THE 5 STEP HORMONE SECRET TO WEIGHT LOSS FOR WOMEN

THE LITTLE-KNOWN SOLUTION TO RESETTING YOUR ADRENAL GLANDS, BOOSTING YOUR METABOLISM, ELEVATING YOUR MOOD, AND LOSING WEIGHT ONCE AND FOR ALL

ELLA RENÉE

indirect, which are incurred as a result of the use of the information contained within this document, including, but not limited to, errors, omissions, or inaccuracies.

CONTENTS

Introduction 7

1. STEP 1: IDENTIFY AND UNDERSTAND 15
YOUR HORMONAL IMBALANCE
What Causes Hormonal Imbalance? 17
Other Things That Can Possibly Cause 35
Hormonal Imbalance
Hormone Imbalance and Cancer 44
Signs of Hormonal Imbalance 46
Why Are Hormones Important for Weight 55
Stability and Health?

2. STEP 2: CORRECT ADRENAL FATIGUE 61
The Role of Adrenal Glands 61
What Hormones do the Adrenal Glands 63
Make?
What is Meant by Adrenal Insufficiency? 69
What Does Adrenal Crisis Mean? 70
What are Adrenal Gland Disorders? 71
Adrenal Fatigue 78
Adrenal Insufficiency 85
How to Fix Adrenal Fatigue and Lower 86
Cortisol Levels

3. STEP 3: GET TO KNOW YOUR 101
SUPERFOODS
Nutrition and Weight Loss 101
33 Superfoods for Weight Loss Success 106
7 Foods to Avoid 110

Vitamins That Assist in Balancing Hormones   112

Foods That Improve Your Mood   115

Additional Benefits of Good Nutrition   118

4. STEP 4: UNDERSTAND NUTRIENT TIMING   127

The Role of Macronutrients   127

Healthy Eating Habits   132

Nutrient Timing - When Should I Eat?   135

5. STEP 5: HOW TO CLEANSE YOUR BODY   139

What Is a Health Cleanse?   139

Benefits of a Health Cleanse   142

How to Detox with a Cleanse?   151

Why Should I Detox?   154

Signs Your Body Needs a Detox   156

How Does Detoxification Work?   165

Other Natural Ways to Detox Your Body   170

How To Tell If Your Liver Detox Is Working?   172

Extra Benefits of Full-Body Cleansing   179

Conclusion   183

Discussion Section   189

Resources   195

INTRODUCTION

Standing in front of the mirror, concealing all bodily flaws, counting all the calories before consuming a favorite food, and manipulating oneself to try a little harder for the perfect shape is the story of every 1 in 4 women worldwide. According to research, there's inevitable and rather exclusive jeopardy of immediate weight gain after the early 30s because women generally have a slower metabolism than men. Obesity becomes inexorable after menopause. Some poor lifestyle choices, such as a substandard diet, affect your metabolism forever. We all know you can't wait further when there's a standard, upscale diet that will solve all your health problems and attenuate the obesity-related trauma.

It's about time someone told you how completely irrelevant and vexatious these theories, or rather myths, actually are. The persistent voices of self-doubt and insecurity post mediocre weight gain will become the most tormenting chapters of your life. It's time to find answers to real questions like, "what do hormones have to do with my mood?", "Can I boost my metabolism?" and "what do I need to know about my adrenal glands before making provisions to lose weight?".

When you first encounter a challenging situation like obesity and irregular weight gain, optimism is vitalizing, and everything seems approachable. Over time the realization of every correlated comorbidity kicks in. There are multiple demonizing factors in your surroundings. You start to notice a vague reorientation of your mental and physical health. In addition, everything you do seems to be enforcing a relapse to phase one of gaining weight. Over time, you become tired of striving for a better shape because of the utmost realization that you'll never be able to fit back into your favorite dress.

Many people believe that weight loss is directly related to happiness, and they could be right if that's what you've been wanting to achieve for the longest time possible. But weight loss isn't just a weekly routine or a monthly schedule; it's a proper journey that takes you to your full potential and makes you the best version of yourself. Still and all, the overwhelming diets that make you cut out everything but a plain bowl of salad and exhausting exercises that may not even burn as many calories as they promise are the biggest, most unnecessary challenges you could take.

While all that may appear like a dead end, it's about time you learned the secrets of balancing your hormones and achieved extended weight-loss results. When you realize that the emotional rollercoaster one embarks on due to the unconventional fat-building, is something you can put aside for good, it opens doors for lifelong lessons about losing weight. Here, you can grasp superior knowledge about accelerating your metabolism to the proper levels and discovering how to keep your weight down for longer periods by doing the bare minimum of effort. Forget about diets and exercises that put you in a bad mood and wreck your self-love.

The well-renowned phrase "comparison is the thief of joy" accurately sums up how immense is the impact of obesity on your life. Those couple of extra pounds trigger overthinking and an inferiority complex that can take months of counseling to overcome. It also becomes a major cause of why many people avert to dietary options, and let's face it, it doesn't work for almost everyone. The proper justification behind that lies in the difference in metabolic rates. A single diet plan found on the internet will only be helpful to 1 out of a hundred people, and that too, only to an extent. So, what distinction lies in the process of resetting patterns of your adrenal glands?

Let's say adrenal glands are responsible for almost every change in your body. It's the hidden, magical ingredient you've left out in your weight loss journey. How many weight loss gurus out there talk about hormonal changes and metabolic rates before moving on to their suggestive dietary plans? To clarify, adrenal glands stimulate hormonal activity in our bodies. These glands have a direct relation to the stress levels in our brains. Weight gain or loss both directly impact the stress levels of our brain. Many people plummet into the abyss of stress-eating whenever they feel the most self-conscious or inferior. Learning how to manage the internal phenomenon in your body will positively impact your health. A slim figure will never make you content with your position in life, but an alleviate mood and a purposeful beginning will have the maximum gratifying effect on your personality. Besides, who wouldn't want to meet the best versions of themselves?

Obesity can be challenging, and more often than not, it's linked to unlikely or concealed diseases that won't show before the aftermath. A little thorough investigation into the depths of this research will leave you with a handful of discoveries about calories, how your body reacts to specific situations, the involvement of adrenal glands in your corporal mechanisms, how to adjust your adrenal glands, get relief from self-invited mood swings, foods to avoid to make this whole scheme a success, and much, much more!

Say goodbye to the days of absolute misery and hope-lessness; where you watched dozens of diet plans crumble before your eyes, exercises that were worth nothing but caused immense fatigue which took you months to get rid of, people telling you to "do more" or rather making nerve-racking comments like "you're already doing enough" which bring you further down, and makes you run in an intense loop that never seems to end and keeps getting worse day by day. It's time for you to plan to try on those eye-catching clothing you'd always wanted to try and feel just how much perfection you've had hidden within yourself, and I'm going to show you exactly how to do that.

Multiple fitness gurus and nutritional science experts will guide you on what worked for them and seek to inspire you with whatever magic trick they've got up their sleeves. But someone like me, who's been studying the science of nutrition for multiple years have practiced helping individuals cross the hurdles and achieve the best version of themselves, will not tell you any story other than sharing good tactics and evident scientific research to help you maintain your weight for longer periods and follow a much healthier lifestyle. While many fitness experts will only focus on a single aspect of the matter, I want to share every single element of my successful practice, coaching, and learning of over 17 years with any soul who's suffering from dealing with the absurdity of this labyrinthine called the human body and whoever wants to learn how to control it for a healthier lifestyle.

Hormonal balance is very close to my heart because I've seen it help numerous people learn how to live a happier life and be content with the process every step of the way. While it may sound like a complex theorem, it's a small web that gradually becomes easier to untangle as you pass all the simple phases of finding hormonal balance. I've helped people achieve that, and I'll help you too. Weight loss is achievable through proper nutrition and breaking barriers to hormonal balance. I realized that I want to share each step to complete hormonal balance that works for everyone struggling to achieve their perfect shape, as many as possible. I'm writing this book out of passion and love for the matter at hand and a benevolent sentiment to anyone it reaches. Your struggle has brought you to this book, don't stop until you're through.

People from the fitness industry often hand you distinct weight loss methods according to your gender. It's time to encompass this dreading discrimination and find absolute bliss by following simple guidelines on how to take control of your body rather than diving right into a diet plan that may or may not work for you. While avoiding a couple of harmful foods can benefit you, it requires an utmost understanding of how your body will reach the absence of that form of food to a long extent. As eager as everyone is to jump right to the bright side and quickly consume information to get to the point where they're in the right shoes, there's much accessible information to learn and practice before. You can't start something if you don't know where you're headed. Rather than shooting bullets into the sky, it's time to take a deep breath and start by identifying the causes of your hormonal imbalance, the signs and symptoms that appear, and how to get your hormones back on track.

CHAPTER 1
STEP 1: IDENTIFY AND UNDERSTAND YOUR HORMONAL IMBALANCE

It's of utmost necessity to understand the gist of hormonal imbalance. Hormonal imbalance is the upsetting discharge or consummation of a particular hormone. Hormones are the channels in your body that drive multiple tissue and organ functions. They are the chemical messengers that keep each organ functioning in a specific pattern. The absence of a single hormone can deprive the organs of their function.

In contrast, an exceeding discharge of the same hormone can make any organ work in overdrive and disrupt metabolisms. While it's completely normal for some hormones to fluctuate throughout your life due to the natural aging process, the main concern arises when the endocrine glands don't respond innately. But what do the endocrine glands have to do with hormonal imbalance?

As the nervous system uses neurotransmitters to get response stimulated across the human body, the endocrine glands utilize hormones for the same process. The endocrine system secretes hormones that travel throughout the bloodstream; an alternation in the secretion of those hormones can affect multiple body functions, including metabolism, mood swings, and appetite, directly related to the person's weight. The endocrine glands do not denote a single pair of glands but a complete network entwined throughout the body. The endocrine system includes adrenal glands found on top of each kidney and plays a vital role in regulating blood pressure, heart rate, and stress response. While other glands in the endocrine system, such as the hypothalamus, stimulate functions like appetite, adrenal glands have a closer relation to the issue at hand- weight loss. An underlying disease may also be why your endocrine system isn't performing innately.

WHAT CAUSES HORMONAL IMBALANCE?

Combating hormonal imbalance requires a thorough understanding of it. There are multiple causes of hormonal imbalance. A handful of diseases can disrupt the performance of your endocrine system. Often, a few changes in diets affect the body negatively. Implementation comes after understanding. You can't jump between different topics without a sequence. That's what most fitness gurus have been making all of their careers. They don't diagnose the problem and may suggest twenty possible solutions to a single issue that you may or may not have. That's why multiple dietary plans do not work for everyone. Hormonal imbalance is sourced through almost anything, so it's compulsory to understand the natural causes first.

Every organism is gifted with a body that responds to internal and external stimuli entirely different from the rest of the organisms. Hence, it determines the importance of understanding what natural causes may have disrupted your hormonal patterns. One must realize that naturally occurring hormonal imbalances are completely involuntary because it's an innate response of your body to a particular situation or change inside the body. Naturally caused imbalances are more challenging to overcome because it's not your lifestyle choices that need alternation. As mentioned earlier, some hormonal imbalance, like reducing the activity of a particular hormone, is completely natural due to the aging factor. Many people stress over a few changes in their body which only adds fuel to hormonal imbalances. Stress is a primary factor of disturbance in adrenal glands and the weight we carry.

Naturally caused hormonal imbalances can be due to the decline in the performance of a particular organ, prolonged treatment of a disease or illness, or, as mentioned earlier, your bodily processes giving in to old age. On the contrary, there are three leading causes of hormonal imbalance directly or indirectly related to your weight loss journey.

1. Stress
2. Dysfunction of thyroid glands.
3. Eating disorders

Stress

The first cause of hormonal imbalance triggers the rest of the causes because stress is the root of multiple detrimental health issues in the human body. When a person feels a particular fear of anything or has been through physical injury or emotional trauma, the endocrine system releases hormones like adrenaline and cortisol in response to the tension and stress levels throughout the human body. While the adrenaline hormone is responsible for many functions, including the racing heartbeat, cortisol is the primary hormone directly linked with carbs, proteins, and fats. But what does a stress-reducing hormone have to do with weight loss?

When the human body experiences stress, the primary innate response of the body is an activation of the pituitary and adrenal gland axis. This activation leads to the secretion of corticotropin or CRF, which results in the production of the cortisol hormone from the pituitary glands. The pituitary gland controls almost all body functions below the brain's hypothalamus. It secretes so many hormones that it's impossible to think it wouldn't play a vital role in relieving stress. So, where is this cortisol hormone secreted?

Cortisol is produced right above the kidneys because it helps reduce inflammation, boosts energy levels within the human body, regulates blood pressure that may rise or fall due to stress, controls sugar levels, and processes the sleep/wake cycle of the human body. Most importantly, it helps the body consume carbs, fats, and proteins. In cases of chronic stress, the cortisol keeps regulating within the bloodstream and triggers various lethal health issues, including digestion problems; it overall causes a hormonal imbalance within the human body.

What are the Consequences of Long-Term Stress?

A little stress every now and then is not something to be worried about. But ongoing, chronic stress can resonate or irritate many serious fitness problems, including:

- Mental health conditions, mainly depression, anxiety, and personality disorders
- Cardiovascular disease, along with heart disease, excessive blood pressure, bizarre heart rhythms, coronary heart attacks, and strokes
- Obesity and other eating disorders
- Menstrual problems
- Sexual dysfunction, such as impotence. Loss of sexual desire in both genders.
- Skin problems; acne, psoriasis, eczema, etc.
- Permanent hair loss and additional hair problems.
- Gastrointestinal problems, such as GERD

(Gastroesophageal reflux disease), gastritis, ulcerative colitis, and irritable colon.

▶ Coronary Diseases

These diseases can be triggered by multiplied blood strain brought on by neither secretion of norepinephrine nor cortical. These ailments include hypertension, tachycardia, and even an increased possibility of having a coronary heart attack or stroke.

▶ Dermatological Disorders

Hormonal and endocrine disruptions caused by stress can cause eruptions on the skin like pimples (from excess sebaceous secretion). Many other dermatological conditions are observed on our skin, such as alopecia, blemishes, eczema, dryness, excessive sweating, and nail weakness because the skin is the primary indicator of our health.

▶ Gastrointestinal Disorders

Increased secretions of gastric juices can cause stomach ulcers, digestive problems, nausea, diarrhea, stomach pain, and even a circumstance known as irritable colon/bowel syndrome.

▶ Respiratory Disorders

Sustained stress makes us more likely to have allergies, sleep apnea (cuts in breathing while napping that limit sleep quality), and asthma.

▶ Muscular and Articulator Problems

Due to the continuous anxiety of the muscles, neck, and lower back, pains, jerks, and contractures are frequent. In addition, this, in turn, motives particular problems.

▶ Headaches and Migraines

Increasing blood strain can purpose meninges (layers that wrap around the brain) to swell and lead to complications. In some severe cases, there's the inconvenience of migraines. The brain is the distinct organ in the human body that doesn't have any pain receptors; therefore, when our head hurts, it is not due to the fact nothing takes place; it is commonly due to the inflammation of the meninges.

▶ Immunological Disorders

The defenses go down if the demanding scenario lasts over time; therefore, you are more likely to get infectious diseases.

▶ Disorders of the Sexual Organs

The intercourse organs may deteriorate due to hormonal imbalances brought about by high stress. This deterioration can lead to changes in menstrual cycles, diminished sexual appetite, irritation, and even infertility in both guys and women.

▶ Problems of Growth

The peak we will attain in our maturity is predetermined genetically; however, in our genes, there is no genuine parent if there is no longer an interval inside which our top may additionally be. The peak we reach inside that range depends on environmental factors, and one of them is stress. It has been tested, that adults who suffered stress during their childhood do now not reach the most height of their interval.

▶ Depression

It has been verified that this sickness is more significant in patients with chronic stress. Stress is the root cause of depression.

▶ Anxiety Disorders

People who suffer from chronic stress in their everyday lives are greater in all likelihood of going through anxiousness disorders because they turn out to be too active in annoying conditions due to the fact of the diabolic mastering process defined above.

▶ Chronic Pain

Some studies have shown that persistent stress produces hyperalgesia (excessive sensitivity to pain) in the internal organs and the somatosensory device and, therefore, is more likely to suffer from persistent pain.

▶ Disorders of Sexual Behavior

High degrees of stress can lead to a sexual conduct sickness referred to as Hypoactive Sexual Desire Disorder. This disorder is more regular in women and entails the innovative loss of sexual desire.

▶ Sleep Disorders

It is frequent for human beings who go through excessive tiers of stress to develop sleep issues such as insomnia. In addition, in the latest study, it has been shown that the ways that human beings have to deal with stress are inefficient.

▶ Eating Disorders

One of the most frequent eating problems in people with stress is Binge Eating Disorder. Episodes of binge eating characterize this sickness, i.e., the man or woman eats an immoderate quantity of meals for very little time and has a feeling of loss of management over what he is doing.

▶ Alzheimer's

Some studies exhibit that stress motivates the untimely aging of key areas of the brain, such as the hypothalamus, and consequently increases the likelihood of growing Alzheimer's disease.

Numerous studies propose that the journey of stress is vital for the onset of acute psychosis. Recent research has proven that this is so; poorly managed disturbing experiences that cause soreness and nervousness can lead to the emergence of psychotic symptoms in persons with a genetic predisposition. In addition, if these persons have experienced a trip of childhood trauma, they are pretty likely to improve psychosis.

▶ Adaptive Disease or Persistent Stress

Persistent stress is a kind of adjustment disorder characterized by an unhealthy emotional and behavioral response to an identifiable and extended stress situation. This disorder appears when the individual undergoes extended stress and does not lift out adaptive responses to that stress.

▶ Irritable Bowel Syndrome

This syndrome is caused without delay through a situation that motives excessive stress or extended stress. The endocrine systems enter the mode of hyperactivity which can motivate an expansion insensitivity in the interior organs, such as the colon or intestine.

▶ Post-Traumatic Stress Disorder

This sickness takes place due to a worrying trip that motives acute stress. There are a lot of conditions that trigger chronic stress situations, such as suffering sexual abuse or witnessing a catastrophe. It does not show up in all human beings who go through this kind of experience; it is more popular to increase if the ride has happened all through the childhood of the man or woman or if he uses strategies that are no longer adaptive to deal with stress.

Dysfunction of Thyroid Glands

The motive behind discussing thyroid glands before balancing hormones for a better shape is that the thyroid gland is responsible for the chemical breakdown of food within the human body's cells. Thyroids are located in the neck, and the hormones produced by the thyroid gland directly relate to digestion. Our brain naturally releases a thyroid-stimulating hormone that can drastically affect our entire body if there's even a mediocre change in its production. The thyroid may secrete specific hormones, but each one of those hormones is essential for a sequenced metabolism. Numerous problems arise due to a thyroid imbalance because two major diseases are linked to these glands.

1. Hyperthyroidism (overactive thyroid glands)
2. Hypothyroidism (underactive thyroid glands)

▶ Hyperthyroidism

When the thyroid glands produce too much of the thyroid hormone, it accelerates the rest of the bodily functions controlled by the thyroid; the blood pressure is increased, and a person diagnosed with thyroid may suffer from inevitable shaking of hands and the rest of the body, perspiration rates increase involuntarily, (in women) there are changes in menstrual cycles; you may experience shorter or lighter periods due to hyperthyroidism. This form of hormonal imbalance is extremely rare. Hyperthyroidism also affects the digestive system-it triggers a sudden change in the body's bowel movements.

▶ Hypothyroidism

Often people have been diagnosed with the low functioning of thyroids, knowns as hypothyroidism, and it messes up how their body responds to normal stimuli. Hypothyroidism is more common than a hyperthyroid condition because it can result from any reason, including increasing age. It is also more common in women. Low thyroid hormone production can deprive the body of many innate combat skills and make the person more vulnerable and prone to many diseases. For instance, a person with hypothyroidism will struggle to combat normal degrees of cold in winter, weight gain, sleeplessness, the spontaneous activity of thyroid glands at irregular hours of the day, increase or decrease in blood flow, etc. It is the most common form of hormonal imbalance and can have dangerous results on your body.

Eating Disorders

Malnutrition roots multiple health problems, and hormonal imbalances are one of them. There are various types of eating disorders, but the subject of attention is how those eating disorders affect the body and trigger a weight gain. Disorders such as anorexia which is a case of self-starvation rather than primary malnutrition, can result in a rapid fall in the production of thyroid and decrease sex drive in humans. Hormones are secreted to store energy the body gains from food, and eating disorders can create multiple hurdles in the way for those hormones and ultimately force them to fail.

For instance, if a person is diagnosed with an eating disorder at the early stages of their growing age, their puberty and growth rate hormones will suffer a massive decline due to low energy consumption for the hormones to stabilize. This type of hormonal imbalance will ultimately decrease the body's development rate and drastically impact bone growth. Eating disorders are directly linked to thyroid problems and correlate with hypothyroidism. Hypothyroidism powered by eating disorders can result in constipation.

Eating disorders have an immense impact on the physical, emotional, and psychological portions of the human body. The healthy image or appearance gradually slumps due to low food consumption. It also upsets hormones responsible for cortisol, which plays a vital role in handling emotions. We already know that thyroid hormones are linked with health, but these hormones also perform a veiled operation of inducing happiness. The negative effects of eating disorders can also impact endorphins that boost our moods. Many hormones go hand in hand with the weight and mood of your body. It ultimately reinforces the importance of learning proper hormonal balance for a healthy and sustainable lifestyle.

Signs that you may have an eating disorder,

Mental and behavioral signs and symptoms may additionally consist of:

- Dramatic weight loss
- Concern about ingesting in public
- Preoccupation with weight, food, calories, fat grams, or dieting
- Complaints of constipation, stomach pain, and other G.I. related issues, lethargy, or excess energy
- excuses to keep away from mealtime
- intense worry of weight gain or being "fat"
- dressing in layers to hide weight loss or remain warm
- Severely limiting and prescribing the amount and kinds of meals consumed
- refusing to consume some foods

- Denying feeling hungry
- Expressing a need to "burn off" calories
- Repeatedly weighing oneself
- patterns of binge ingesting and purging
- Developing rituals around food
- Excessively exercising
- Cooking foods for others without eating
- Missing menstrual periods (in human beings who would commonly menstruate)

Physical symptoms may also include:

- Stomach cramps and other gastrointestinal symptoms
- Difficulty concentrating
- The atypical lab takes a look at outcomes (anemia, low thyroid levels, low hormone levels, low potassium, low blood phone counts, slow coronary heart rate)
- Dizziness
- Fainting
- Feeling cold all the time
- Sleep irregularities
- Menstrual irregularities
- Calluses throughout the tops of the finger joints (a sign of inducing vomiting)

- dry skin
- dry, thin nails
- Thinning hair
- Muscle weakness
- poor wound healing
- poor immune system characteristic

Multiple eating disorders like anorexia nervosa in which people are very underweight as a result of severe weight-reduction plans or immoderate exercise. Similarly, those who suffer from bulimia nervosa have a 'normal weight' but have cycles of uncontrollable overeating. During this time, they eat large quantities of food while feeling out of control and powerless to cease (bingeing), accompanied by making themselves ailing after foods or abusing laxatives (purging) to make up for the meals eaten. In contrast, humans with a binge-eating disease have available episodes of uncontrollable binge eating however do not strive to make up for the binges through vomiting, fasting, or over-exercising. As a result, humans with a binge-eating disease frequently become obese.

How Metabolism Is Affected by Eating Disorders

The set of chemical reactions occurring within the human body that enables it to grow, keep power ranges, and respond to the surroundings are known as metabolisms. Several hormones are concerned with regulating the body's metabolism, many of which are severely affected by the way of ingesting disorders. These hormonal modifications are a great response to starvation and will serve to keep energy. When a consuming disorder begins in the early years, it can alter the hormones concerned in puberty and growth. Puberty might also be delayed, and bones may also fail to grow, leading to a small increase and brittle bones (osteoporosis) later in life.

Eating issues can additionally lead to low levels of thyroid hormones (hypothyroidism), and human beings will often feel cold and whinge with constipation. Dry Skin is another emerging symptom of eating disorders.

▶ Impact on Stress Hormones

Eating disorders significantly affect the production of stress hormones, which include cortisol, growth hormone, and noradrenaline. These hormones are usually launched in greater amounts at points of high stress. The fluctuation of stress hormones due to eating disorders leads to sleep problems, feelings of anxiety, depression, and panic. Similarly, there is a sturdy bodily response which includes an amplification in heart rate and respiration.

▶ Effects on Fertility and Pregnancy

Eating disorders ordinarily affect younger humans at what would otherwise be the height of their reproductive lives. Unhealthy eating styles can lead to modifications in reproductive hormones responsible for retaining regular periods, intercourse drive, healthful hearts, and sturdy bones. As a result, some girls will have irregular periods, some will cease having them all together, and some might also go through infertility. Men, on the different hand, may also lose their sex power or have erectile problems. This is, again, the body's response to an attempt to retain electricity and stop reproduction in a ravenous individual. Hormones return to normal levels once consumption is returned to normal.

In the few cases where being pregnant does occur, ingesting issues also influence reproductive hormones all through pregnancy, affecting both the mother and child. Some research recommends that females with consumption problems are at a greater danger of issues around the time of pregnancy, together with the need for a cesarean section, postnatal depression, miscarriage, tricky delivery, and untimely birth. But if you recover from eating disorders, it has no impact on your pregnancies in the latter.

▶ Eating Disorders and Obesity

In binge-eating disorder, compulsive overeating typically leads to obesity. Obesity, in turn, causes several scientific complications such as high cholesterol levels, diabetes, coronary heart disease, gallstones, gout, and certain kinds of cancer. Obesity also causes an expansion in hormone tiers that encourages the build-up of body fat, hence making it even harder to lose weight. Treatment focuses on psychological exchange (for example, addressing the emotional reasons why anybody feels they have to overeat) and behavioral changes, such as healthy eating and ordinary exercise.

OTHER THINGS THAT CAN POSSIBLY CAUSE HORMONAL IMBALANCE

▶ Pregnancy:

This is one of the more apparent causes of hormone imbalance. The degrees of several different hormones exchanged throughout pregnancy can trigger multiple health issues. Luckily the hormonal imbalances linked to being pregnant are transient and resolve some time after the child is born. But they're very hard to overcome at a rapid rate.

Certain hormonal imbalances can affect your capacity to get pregnant. Hormones adjust physical features such as maintaining your regular menstrual cycle, preparing your body for pregnancy, defending unfertilized eggs, and ovulation. If just one of the methods essential for being pregnant is out of balance, it will become harder for you to conceive. Hormonal imbalance can even lead to infertility.

Once you are pregnant, hormones continue to play an essential role. Pregnancy hormones hold the fitness of your baby, manage its rate of growth, and even set off the labor process. As a result, hormonal imbalance in the course of being pregnant can motive troubles together with gestational diabetes, preeclampsia, high or low delivery weight, or even miscarriage. Infertility can be a very traumatizing experience and a leading cause of hormonal imbalance; PCOS can become the issue.

The hormonal imbalance that occurs during this condition interferes with ovulation. You can't get pregnant if you're no longer ovulating. Pregnancy is still viable if you have PCOS. If your doctor recommends it, losing weight can make a huge difference in your fertility. Prescription medicines are also available to stimulate ovulation and extend your possibility of turning pregnant. PCOS can cause issues for both you and your baby. It ultimately leads to:

1. miscarriage
2. gestational diabetes
3. preeclampsia
4. cesarean delivery
5. high beginning weight
6. admission to and time spent in the neonatal intensive care unit

Key Hormones That Affect Fertility

While it's actual that we have lots of distinctive hormones coursing through our bodies, solely a few come into play when we're attempting to conceive. Below are some of the key fertility hormones you may want to get acquainted with if you suspect a hormone imbalance may be affecting your capacity to get pregnant. You can get a perspective of these hormones by getting a hormone check.

- FSH is one of the most crucial hormones for normal fertilization. FSH, or follicle-stimulating hormone, is responsible for retaining cycle regularity and producing healthy eggs to be fertilized.

- LH, or luteinizing hormone, is another fertility hormone essential for a normal pregnancy; it's the hormone that you can easily measure in at-home ovulation predictor kits (OPKs). That's why many women can instantly recall this one. LH is the hormone that issues an indicator for your body to release an egg because it is prepared to be fertilized.

- AMH, also known as the anti-Mullerian hormone, is accountable for preserving your physique's immature eggs. It is the hormone that measures your ovarian reserve. It means it calculates how many eggs you have left.

- Progesterone is a critical participant in making ready the physique for being pregnant and assisting a new pregnancy to continue. Often when a woman suffers repeated miscarriages, plummeting progesterone ranges are the culprit.

- Prolactin If you are questioning that this hormone is the one that handles milk production, you're correct! But it is additionally a key player in making sure your cycle stays regular, which is vital when attempting to conceive.

- T3 and T4 - Many girls don't comprehend this. However, these thyroid hormones have a major influence on the ability to get pregnant. Studies by various doctors indicate that the thyroid gland, woman's reproductive organs, and adrenal glands are intricately connected. Turning pregnant can be a challenge if there is an issue with both the thyroid and the adrenals. In many cases, when the thyroid hormones are back to normal, many women find it easier to get pregnant.

▶ Breastfeeding:

Some of the hormonal troubles that pregnant females ride will become less great after they begin and recover. But, breastfeeding an infant can also affect hormone levels. There are two hormones without delay associated with breastfeeding: prolactin and oxytocin. Breastfeeding can also affect progesterone because ladies who breastfeed may also have irregular menstrual cycles or no cycle.

▶ Polycystic Ovary Syndrome (PCOS):

This is a common hormonal disease among ladies of reproductive age. Hormonal imbalances create issues in multiple parts of your body, including the ovaries, which release an egg to be fertilized each month as a part of a healthy and accurate menstrual cycle. With PCOS, the egg may no longer advance as it ought to, or it may also no longer be released all through ovulation as it must be.

Primary ovarian insufficiency or untimely ovarian failure. It occurs when the ovaries quit generally functioning before age forty. The ovaries cease producing the everyday quantity of estrogen or release eggs for ovulation. This frequently leads to infertility. Some of the symptoms of PCOS include:

- Irregular menstrual cycle. Women with PCOS can also leave out durations or have fewer periods (fewer than eight in a year). Or, their durations might also come every 21 days or extra often. Some women with PCOS give up having menstrual periods.
- There is too much hair on the face, chin, or parts of the physique where men usually have

hair. This is called "hirsutism." Hirsutism affects up to 70% of ladies with PCOS.

- Acne on multiple areas of the body, especially the chest, upper back, and face.
- Male-pattern baldness; thinning of hair
- Weight gain or situation in which you're losing weight
- Darkening of skin, specifically along neck creases, in the groin, and under breasts or chest area.
- Skin tags, minor flaps of pores, and skin in the armpits or neck area

▶ Diabetes:

Diabetes can throw off the stability of hormones in your body. Diabetes takes place when the pancreas no longer produces sufficient amounts of the hormone insulin. Or, the physique can't use the insulin the pancreas makes. Insulin helps metabolize the sugar we devour into strength for our cells. If there are no longer sufficient amounts or if the physique isn't properly used, then there will be too much sugar in the blood.

The Connection Between Diabetes and Hormone Imbalance

There's a two-way hyperlink between diabetes and hormonal imbalance. Diabetes can develop through hormonal imbalance or vice versa. Your pancreas produces the hormone insulin. Insulin is absorbed from your blood by your fat, muscle, and liver cells for energy. Insulin additionally aids different metabolic approaches in your body.

With type two diabetes, your physique develops insulin resistance. Your pancreas works tougher to produce greater insulin to reduce multiplied blood glucose levels. However, it can't hold up. In many cases, the victim has uncontrolled high blood pressure. The two-way aspect of diabetes is that it's linked to hormonal imbalance and can be a prime cause in most cases.

For instance, menopausal hormonal modifications influence your blood sugar level, and postmenopausal ladies can have drastic fluctuations and extra blood sugar if they have diabetes. The weight acquired related to menopause would also require that your diabetes remedy be changed. At the same time, decreasing hormone degrees can disturb your sleep, making it more challenging to manage blood sugar levels.

Women with diabetes might also trip more sexual dysfunction than usual because the circumstance is related to injury of the cells in the vaginal lining. Men experience the same problems when their bodies produce less testosterone, decreased muscle mass, and a slow intercourse drive. But many human beings don't know that lowered testosterone also contributes to insulin resistance.

▶ Tumors and most Cancer Treatments:

If a tumor is on or near a gland in the endocrine system, it can affect the hormones that the gland produces and delivers. This is real in both benign (non-cancerous) and cancerous tumors. Also, most cancer treatments like chemotherapy or Hormone disruptors.

Hormone disruptors are external factors that include chemical compounds or houses that can affect your body's endocrine system. Some of these disruptors are environmental, and some are things we consume. Some things that might also be hormone disruptors encompass foods, personal care products, cleaning supplies, food containers, drinking water, and a variety of medications. Radiation can also affect hormone levels too.

HORMONE IMBALANCE AND CANCER

The fluctuation and stability of hormones can be influenced by employing a range of factors. There should be a natural change in hormone manufacturing due to monthly cycles or modifications such as age or pregnancy. A hormone imbalance may be caused by a fitness condition. In many cases, medication also seems to be the source. For instance, testosterone can be produced from cholesterol, forcing a deadly prostate cancer in men.

In addition, estrogen is recognized to pressure endometrial cancer, some types of breast cancers, and a quantity of different gynecologic cancers. Excess estrogen might also result from prescribed tablets, but greater likely, your very own body produces it. A granulosa cell-phone tumor of the ovary can produce estrogen.

Obesity is a principal aspect of many cancers. Excessive fat tissue can create estrogen. It can also convert androgen into estrogen. The cumulative impact of estrogen over the lifespan is hazardous for these cancers. Another risk factor would be starting menstruation at an earlier age. On the different hand, for the duration of pregnancy, a woman's estrogen levels are lower, so pregnancies have a bit of a defensive impact against estrogen-driven cancers. Birth control tablets and intrauterine units are regularly protective against hormone-driven cancers.

A Hormone Sensitive Cancer:

Hormone-sensitive cancer, or hormone-dependent cancer, is a kind of cancer based on a hormone for the increase and survival. Examples include breast cancer, which is structured on estrogens like estradiol, and prostate cancer, which is dependent on androgens like testosterone.

Hormones play essential roles in our body; they're also disadvantages in some types of cancers which utilize and promote some tumors to grow and spread, which are so-called hormone-sensitive or hormone-dependent cancer. Hormone-sensitive cancer, or hormone-dependent cancer, is a kind of cancer that is established on a hormone for boom and survival. If a tumor is hormone-sensitive, its abilities there are distinct proteins known as receptors on the cells surface. When the hormone binds to the matched receptor, it increases and spreads cancer cells.

SIGNS OF HORMONAL IMBALANCE

Hormonal imbalance isn't a term assigned to a single abnormality leading to disease. It can come in several forms, and once in a while, the signs and symptoms are almost undetectable. Here are some symptoms of hormonal imbalance that are correlated to weight gain.

- Weight gain
- Mood swings
- Irregular period
- Low sex drive
- Infertility
- Insomnia
- Bloating

▶ Weight Gain

Hormones play an integral position in preserving many critical chemical processes within the body. Because hormones play a big part in regulating your metabolism and how your body uses energy, hormonal imbalance can cause weight gain. Hormonal issues that affect your hormone tiers — such as Cushing's Syndrome — can lead to weight gain. Hypothyroidism is another situation that disrupts hormone levels and can lead to weight gain.

Other elements such as age can also lead to a hormonal imbalance that motivates an amplification in weight. Hormonal imbalance can interfere with healthy meal cues and regulate energy levels within the body. This can sooner or later lead to tremendous weight acquisition and obesity. Research indicates that hormonal imbalance can have a considerable influence on metabolism. For example, a frequent symptom of PCOS is a lack of insulin sensitivity. Insulin regulates blood sugar, so abnormal or decreased insulin sensitivity can cause weight gain.

Many believe that a healthy food regimen and everyday workout must lead to a wholesome weight. But the scale stays the same for many who rely on their efforts in the gym. In some cases, regardless of perfect weight loss efforts, a person's weight increases. For people residing with hormonal imbalances, their metabolisms work against them. This results in many clinical problems, including weight gain. Even when dieting and exercising regularly, people with hormonal issues continue to have unexplained weight gain, but why?

Another necessary characteristic of cortisol is that it manages how your physique uses carbohydrates, fats, and proteins. When cortisol tiers rise, so does your insulin rate. High cortisol triggers thyroid functions, weight fluctuations, and decreased metabolism rates. When cortisol rises, the body grows to be insensitive to insulin. The result is unexplained weight gain, excessive blood sugar levels, and the development of type two diabetes in extreme cases.

High levels of estrogen cause extra fatty tissue growth, and your fat cells, in turn, make more estrogen, so it's a vicious cycle. This excess fat is commonly found around the belly because estrogen dictates where the body distributes fat. Hence, you know that estrogen with progesterone is where you pick a start.

▶ Mood swings

There are many possible causes of mood swings. However, a hormonal imbalance is at the root. This may be because of fluctuating hormone tiers during the menstrual cycle or the duration up to menopause (peri-menopause). It may also be an imbalance influenced by various environmental factors. There is comfort in understanding that your moods are triggered by a fluctuation or imbalance in your hormones.

Patients describe mood swings as feeling "out of control." They were also highly sensitive to matters that normally wouldn't affect them. For many women, mood swings are a product of anxiety, a tendency closer to a depressive mood, insomnia, or feeling over-whelmed. These problems can affect intellectual and physical well-being. The hormone with the most power over mood swings is estrogen. Estrogen influences mood in a few distinctive ways; however, one of the most vital methods is its relationship with serotonin.

Serotonin is a neurotransmitter whose principal accountability is in influencing mood. Fluctuating sero-tonin levels will occur as mood swings, and estrogen influences how tons of serotonin is produced. Low estrogen levels frequently lead to low or inconsistent serotonin levels, which can be a foremost cause of mood swings. Low estrogen can also lead to brain fog symptoms, disturbing sleeping schedules, hot flashes, headaches, and memory issues.

Estrogen also helps shield the brain and nerves from damage, controls the levels of other vital mood-related neurotransmitters, which include dopamine and norepinephrine, and enlarges feel-good endorphins. It's normal for estrogen levels to alter through the distinctive ranges of a woman's life. Estrogen ranges alternate at multiple points of our menstrual cycles to trigger pre and post-menopause ovulation. No matter what stage of life you're in, the key to a healthy lifestyle is to find as much balance as possible.

▶ Irregular Periods

Irregular periods occur much less than 24 days after the previous cycle or no more than 38 days apart. The cycle fluctuates between 24 to 38 days. Suppose your cycle length changes more than 20. days every month, that's also considered an irregular period. It's normal to have one or two irregular periods annually. But if you have more than that, then it may take a thorough overview of the functioning patterns of your hormones to get your body back on track.

All of these issues are rooted in hormonal imbalance, and there is a lot you can do to regain hormonal balance naturally. The strategy is to provide your body with the assistance it needs to make and balance its hormones while reducing the load on your endocrine system. The two main hormones that can upset your menstrual cycles are estrogen and progesterone.

▶ Low Sex Drive

The hormonal imbalances in perimenopause, menopause, and postmenopause typically result in women declining sexual desire or low libido. The major hormone culprits are progesterone, testosterone, and estrogen. Progesterone naturally ceases to produce in perimenopause, resulting in estrogen dominance, which causes low libido in women.

In terms of libido, testosterone in females increase sexual response and orgasms. As a result, low testosterone causes a loss of libido. Experts say that loss of sexual desire or low sex drive may be associated with decreased estrogen, progesterone, or testosterone levels, frequently in menopause. Low libido in women is the most frequent sexual complaint made by females – up to 30/40%. Even younger females feel the impact of a hormonal imbalance on their sex life.

Levels of necessary sex hormones like DHEA and testosterone may decrease in our 20s, causing a complex hormonal imbalance. But it's also considered natural to some extent as well. Besides low sex drive, perimenopause triggers mood swings, weight gain, difficulty sleeping, fatigue, and other symptoms.

▶ Infertility

Infertility can be a heartbreaking experience, but sometimes the solutions are easier than you realize. One of the many things that can affect your possibility of getting pregnant is an imbalance of hormones. Endocrinological abnormalities and hormonal imbalances need to be cured right to treat infertility in a person. Couples undergoing surrogation or assisted fertility methods should also have their hormonal imbalances examined. Hormonal infertility is easily handled and cured when you locate its roots.

Over-secretion of Prolactin leads to ovulatory disorders. These glandular problems disrupt the hormonal balance in the human body. Prolactin is responsible for producing milk in the female body, but its imbalance can impede the process of ovulation. Excessive production of Prolactin can cause anovulation, an incomplete ovulation cycle in the body, which triggers the production of androgens, or male hormones. As a result, the estrogen is reduced in the female physique and motivates difficulties in the ovulation process.

▶ Insomnia

Getting good sleep is one of the most crucial phenomena that help the human body stay healthy and aid your immune system. But for human beings dealing with adrenal fatigue and insomnia, or any different type of continual fatigue, the notion of restful sleep feels like a passing dream. Stressed adrenal glands and inconsistent sleep patterns will wreck your daily life routines. If you struggle to fall or remain asleep, you may have underlying troubles such as insomnia.

Hormone imbalance, insomnia, and adrenal fatigue are all correlated. It starts from adrenal fatigue in the body, throwing your hormones off balance; insomnia and other bodily dysfunctions follow. One of the essential hormones of the human body, cortisol, and sleep, works together for multiple reasons. Studying the importance of cortisol in different metabolic processes of your body will allow you to see how connected your hormones and insomnia are.

▶ Bloating

Bloating is one of the symptoms that everyone undeniably hates. For some people, bloating can be solved in a quick matter of what they're eating or not. It helps prevent them from feeling the discomfort and embarrassment that can come with severe bloat. For others, it is a period-related symptom that pops up a month or so and makes their denim suit tighter, and they will feel as if there's a balloon in their abdomen. But there are different reasons you may feel bloated, including hormonal imbalance. Comprehending bloating as a hormone imbalance is the most effective way to avoid that uncomfortable bloat forever.

Estrogen and progesterone are the most important sex hormones in females. If bloating is a monthly occurrence, a predictable section of your menstrual cycle, you can probably blame it on estrogen and progesterone. As these hormones fluctuate, they can influence the digestive tract. In addition, high estrogen degrees can lead to water retention in the body, which causes the feeling of bloating. Likewise, when progesterone is high, meals may take a slower experience through your intestine, resulting in bloating, which is usually the case in the period after ovulation.

Another reason for your consistent bloating could be stress, specifically your "stress hormone," cortisol. When you're continuously under stress from the everyday pressures of life, this survival-mode response of cortisol can backfire. Digestion becomes less of a priority for your body, leading to slower ingestion through your gastrointestinal machine and consequent bloating. High cortisol degrees can mess with your microbiome or the microorganism in your gut, leading to belly problems like gas, cramping, and bloating.

WHY ARE HORMONES IMPORTANT FOR WEIGHT STABILITY AND HEALTH?

If you're experiencing problems with putting weight on too easily or having a hard time losing it, you should be aware of hormonal imbalance's effects on weight stability. They might be a huge factor in the problem, or they might be causing it entirely. Hormonal imbalances could make your weight loss journey impossible.

Hormones are involved with every aspect of health, including growth, development, emotions, appetite, and metabolism. This is why when your body releases too little or too much of a single hormone, it impacts your health and, in this case - body weight. This is what's known as hormonal dysregulation. Some hormones stimulate hunger, making you want to eat more. While others send signals to your body that you've had enough. Hormonal dysregulation in appetite control would lead to gaining or losing weight significantly. Mainly hormones like Ghrelin, the "Hunger Hormone," Motilin, NPY, and AgRp are the ones that stimulate food intake in your body. They are part of a series of steps in the nervous system and endocrine to develop hunger.

As a part of metabolism, fat storage and breakdown are also strictly controlled by specific hormones in the body. They regulate energy expenditure and even the amount of calories your body burns in a single day. Fluctuations in certain areas around the body may cause body fat to accumulate there. For instance, when the thyroid gland becomes overactive and releases an excess of thyroid hormone, it forces the body to burn more calories. This is hyperthyroidism, which we've previously talked about.

1. Leptin: a fat hormone that has been thoroughly researched in recent years, has produced weight loss in many organisms by increasing their metabolism and safely decreasing their appetite. Leptin is among the few major hormones that affect your weight.

2. Insulin: it's the main storage hormone that is the most important one to consider when it comes to weight loss and weight gain. Insulin is secreted in small amounts throughout the day and larger amounts after meals.

- But that's only in healthy individuals; insulin resistance, which causes your cells to stop responding to insulin, is a fairly common health condition for many other people.
- This condition causes high blood sugar and is generally linked to obesity which invites major conditions like type-2 diabetes and heart disease.

3. Cortisol: Known as the stress hormone, was essential for humans during the old ages when survival wasn't guaranteed for everyone, but it's produced more often than needed in the current era. Cortisol is released into your bloodstream whenever your body or mind believes it's under stress. These days, people get stressed over not-so-significant matters, making our bodies create more cortisol than the optimal amount.

Now, you may be familiar with how cortisol links to weight gain. Do you ever notice how people eat more, especially when stressed? Countless studies have shown that cortisol levels are associated with overeating and faster weight gain. Countless hunger and satiety hormones perform the function of appetite control, including,

Hunger hormones

1. Ghrelin
Sends hunger signals to the brain and promotes food absorption.

2. Motilin
Stimulates movement of digestive organs.

3. Neuropeptide Y
NPY plays an integral role in managing stress and anxiety.

4. Agouti-related protein
AgRP increases appetite and decreases metabolism.

Satiety hormones

1. Cholecystokinin
Stimulates pancreas function.

2. Glucagon type peptide-1
Lowers glucose levels in the blood.

3. Pancreatic peptide YY
Stimulates food digestion, gut motility, and insulin secretion.

4. Obestatin
Reduces food intake and positively influences body weight gain.

In addition, the continuous mention of adrenal glands has you thinking, what role do they play in hormonal stability and weight loss?

CHAPTER 2

STEP 2: CORRECT ADRENAL FATIGUE

THE ROLE OF ADRENAL GLANDS

The first thing you need to know about the adrenal glands is where to find them- which would be at the top of each kidney. The hormones in these glands manage the immune system, blood pressure, metabolism, and stress response in the human body. Adrenal glands produce about 150 hormones that regulate different functions in your body. Right now, you might be wondering about how adrenal glands are even remotely related to your condition, but a little preview would just put things in perspective.

One hormone that's name gets thrown around here, and there occasionally is adrenaline, which initiates the fight or flight response in the brain. That's why it's also called a stress hormone. It helps you decide how to combat difficult situations or avoid them entirely. Another hormone, cortisol, is another essential hormone that will reset the course of your bodily functions once you learn how to master its control.

But before that, here's a little preview of the role of adrenal glands in the body.

Anatomy of the Adrenal Glands

The adrenal glands are the two triangular-shaped organs located at the top of the kidney and comprise a total length of 1.5 inches. The adrenal glands consist of two parts:

The adrenal cortex—the outer section of the gland—produces hormones that are crucial for the body, like cortisol, which helps regulate metabolism and helps your physique stress response, and aldosterone (which helps manage blood pressure).

The adrenal medulla—the inner phase of the gland—produces nonessential hormones, like Adrenaline (which helps your body react to stress).

What do Adrenal Glands do?

Adrenal glands are present in the body to produce essential hormones for our health. For instance,

The adrenal cortex produces hormones that are responsible for stimulating sexual desires and responses (androgens, estrogens), salt concentrations in the blood (aldosterone), and sugar stability (cortisol).

The adrenal medulla produces hormones concerned with the fight-or-flight response. It produces hormones like catecholamines or adrenaline.

The Adrenal Medulla and Cortex produce different hormones responsible for distinct functions throughout the human body. While both of these glands are the size of a fortune cookie, each consists of a medulla (middle of the gland) surrounded by the cortex.

WHAT HORMONES DO THE ADRENAL GLANDS MAKE?

The adrenal glands produce hormones including, Adrenaline, noradrenaline, cortisol, and aldosterone.

- Adrenaline and noradrenaline are secreted as a stress response. They make the heart beat faster, transport blood to muscle mass, and motivate other modifications in the body that prepare it to combat distressing situations.
- Cortisol does many things, including influencing metabolism to utilize energy, altering blood sugar stages, and slowing down the immune system.
- Aldosterone plays a section in controlling blood pressure.
- The adrenal glands also produce susceptible sex hormones that tour the testes or ovaries, the place they are converted into testosterone or estrogen.

Adrenal Gland Hormones

1. Epinephrine or Adrenaline:
This hormone rapidly responds to stress by triggering the heart rate and elevating glucose tiers in the blood.

2. Norepinephrine or Noradrenaline:
This hormone works with epinephrine as a reaction to the stress-induced in the body. Its

important feature is to prepare the brain and the body for action against induced stress.

3. Hydrocortisone:
It is commonly called cortisol or a steroid hormone. It is used to regulate body functions like the conversion of fats and carbohydrates to energy and manages the metabolic processes.

4. Corticosterone:
This hormone works with hydrocortisone to manipulate the immune response and prevents inflammatory reactions.

The Function of the Adrenal Medulla

We have all experienced that incredible panic or a sudden nervousness when something happens abruptly, and we get scared. Suddenly, you can feel tingling sensations and experience thoughts of either avoiding the situation or preparing for combat.

There are the "fight-or-flight" symptoms precipitated by the sudden launch of adrenaline from our adrenal glands. Adrenaline generically can be broken down into two hormones that the adrenal medulla produces: epinephrine and norepinephrine.

Adrenal Medulla Hormones

The dissimilarity between the adrenal cortex and medulla is that the adrenal medulla does not perform any vital functions inside the human body. One may think that it's not slightly necessary for existence either, but that doesn't mean the adrenal medulla isn't an integral part of the endocrine system or plays no important role in hormonal balance in your body.

The adrenal medulla hormones are a reaction to the stimulation of the sympathetic nervous system, which takes place when you're stressed. As such, the adrenal medulla helps deal with physical and emotional stress.

Hormones secreted by the adrenal medulla are:

The important hormones secreted by using the adrenal medulla include epinephrine (adrenaline) and norepinephrine (noradrenaline), which have correlated functions in the body.

The Function of the Adrenal Cortex

The adrenal cortex produces a handful of hormones quintessential for fluid and electrolyte (salt) equilibrium in the body, like cortisol and aldosterone. The adrenal cortex is responsible for making small quantities of sex hormones. The three layers of the adrenal cortex are:

- Microscopic view of the adrenal cortex: The layers of the adrenal gland cortex, zona glomerulosa (ZG), zona fasciculata (ZF), and zona reticularis (ZR), are accountable for producing aldosterone, cortisol, and sex steroid hormone.

- The zona glomerulosa (ZG) is the most superficial layer of the adrenal cortex, and it produces the hormone aldosterone and some small quantities of progesterone (a sex hormone). The mineralocorticoid aldosterone is produced here.

- The zona fasciculata (ZF) is the middle part of the adrenal cortex, mainly producing cortisol.

- The zona reticularis (ZR) is the adrenal cortex's inner region adjoining the adrenal medulla. Functions of the zona reticularis are the maintenance of cholesterol for steroidogenesis and the secretion of sex hormones like estrogen and testosterone.

Adrenal Cortex Hormones

The adrenal cortex produces two major corporations of corticosteroid hormones: glucocorticoids and mineralocorticoids. The hypothalamus and pituitary gland bring on the release of glucocorticoids. Mineralocorticoids are mediated with the aid of alerts caused by the kidney.

The hypothalamus produces corticotropin-releasing hormone (CRH), which stimulates the pituitary gland to launch adrenocorticotropic hormone (ACTH). These hormones, in turn, alert the adrenal glands to produce corticosteroid hormones.

Glucocorticoids launched by the adrenal cortex include:

- Hydrocortisone: Commonly called cortisol, regulates how the body converts fats, proteins, and carbohydrates to energy. It helps alter blood strain and cardiovascular function.
- Corticosterone: This hormone works with hydrocortisone to manage the immune response and suppress inflammatory reactions.

The principal mineralocorticoid is aldosterone, which keeps the proper stability of salt and water while helping manipulate blood pressure. A 1/3 class of hormones is released by using the adrenal cortex, called sex steroids or sex hormones. However, their impact is usually undermined by the higher production of hormones like estrogen and testosterone launched through the ovaries or testes.

WHAT IS MEANT BY ADRENAL INSUFFICIENCY?

Adrenal insufficiency is known as the inability of the adrenal glands to produce an adequate amount of cortisol or aldosterone. It happens because the adrenal layer or cortex is destroyed. This occurs most regularly when you have an autoimmune disorder that forces your body to assault the glands. It can also be triggered by tumors, tuberculosis, and other kinds of infections. There are two types of adrenal insufficiency, and the above described is known as primary adrenal insufficiency.

Secondary adrenal insufficiency is relevantly more prominent and easily occurred than the elemental form. It occurs because you don't have enough adreno-corticotropin (ACTH), the hormone secreted by the pituitary gland. If your pituitary doesn't make sufficient ACTH, your adrenal glands don't make sufficient cortisol.

Secondary adrenal insufficiency most often occurs when you have been taking glucocorticoids (like prednisone) for a prolonged amount of time and then stop too quickly as an alternative than tapering down gradually. It can also increase due to tumors in the pituitary glands pressing on the ordinary pituitary cells or from surgical treatment or radiation to the pituitary gland.

WHAT DOES ADRENAL CRISIS MEAN?

An adrenal crisis is a hazardous clinical emergency. It happens when there's an extreme lack of cortisol in your body. Adrenal crisis is the most severe form of adrenal insufficiency. An adrenal disaster can be life-threatening.

Symptoms of adrenal disaster include:

- A severe ache in your body that comes on quickly.
- Bouts of vomiting and diarrhea.
- Weakness.
- Confusion and loss of consciousness.

- Low blood glucose.
- Low blood pressure.

People suffering from adrenal insufficiency must continuously carry an injectable structure of glucocorticoid medicine with them. They should also wear some kind of medical alert ring with that information. These conditions cannot be concealed with any kind of sugar coating. People that suffer from adrenal insufficiency often stay around other people that know how to deliver emergency injections and provide extreme care in case of any inconvenience. Other hormone imbalances and symptoms can manifest with adrenal disorders. These encompass having too much potassium (hyperkalemia) or no longer ample sodium (hyponatremia) in your blood.

WHAT ARE ADRENAL GLAND DISORDERS?

Adrenal gland problems run the gamut from causation and treatment. However, they can severely inhibit an individual from thriving physically and mentally. The following adrenal gland problems include:

- **Addison's disease.** This adrenal insufficiency disease is caused by underproducing adrenal glands and is generally precipitated via an existing autoimmune ailment like HIV, Lupus, and type I diabetes. The failure to produce enough quantities of hormones, inclusive of cortisol and aldosterone, results in multiple drastic symptoms, including fatigue, nausea, and muscle weakness. It eventually leads to an Addisonian disease or adrenal crisis – a life-threatening state of affairs that requires immediate cure from a hospital.

- **Cushing's disease.** Unlike Addison's disease, Cushing's is induced by the overproduction of hormones inside the adrenal glands. They send a good deal of cortisol hormone directly into the bloodstream. The symptoms include irregular or extreme obesity, high blood pressure, excessive facial hair or hair growth in absurd areas of the body (areas with minimal to no hair), and irregular menstrual cycles. Victims of this disease also grow susceptible to bruising. These signs and symptoms can sincerely deter from high first-class of lifestyles and require a professional diagnosis, monitoring, and treatment.

- **Adrenal incidentaloma**. Caused with the aid of loads or tumors observed on the adrenal glands. It causes an abruption of hormones-producing single or multiple hormones in outrageous amounts. Surgery is the primary to eliminate them.

- **Pheochromocytomas.** Those with this adrenal disease go through tumors that develop in the medulla, leading to the overproduction of epinephrine and norepinephrine. An extra quantity of these hormones causes high blood pressure, which ultimately triggers coronary heart attacks or a heart stroke.

- **Pituitary tumors.** These are located at the base of the brain. The pituitary gland is also accountable for releasing hormones into our bodies. Certain hormones, which include adrenocorticotropic, set off the adrenal glands to pump cortisol into the bloodstream. A lack of conversation between the pituitary gland and the adrenal glands because benign or cancerous tumors can throw the complete device out of whack.

- **Adrenal gland suppression.** Steroid usage regularly leads to the suppression of adrenal glands. Since steroids mimic cortisol, the adrenal glands can be notified to launch less of this cortisol. When steroid remedy is halted without delay, the adrenal glands may no longer acquire the message to take up the advent of cortisol. A hormone imbalance can make certain and proceed for weeks or even months until the adrenal glands stabilize again.

What are the Signs of Adrenal Disorders?

Adrenal problems can present themselves in a wide variety of ways. Symptoms may additionally vary relying on the person and preexisting conditions but regularly encompass the following:

- Weight loss
- Muscle weakness
- Fatigue
- Darkening of the skin
- Headaches
- Nausea
- Vomiting
- Diarrhea
- Craving salty foods
- Mouth sores
- Abdominal ache

- Constipation

While signs and symptoms vary, there are particular dominant signs and symptoms that convey something may also be wrong with your adrenal glands. Those include:

- Abdominal pain and weight loss. Hormones produced in the adrenal glands manipulate our appetites and food processing. When they are overactive or underproduced, this can lead to digestive troubles and hinder your physique from gleaning the vitamins it needs from meal sources.
- High blood pressure. While this symptom can signify a broad range of ailments, it is specific to adrenal issues when paired with low sodium levels, headaches, and facial flushing. Overproduction of hormones can throw off the careful balance of water and salt in the bloodstream, sending sky-high blood strain.
- Fatigue and weakness. These signs of Addison's ailment are unique and may sign an underlying problem that needs immediate attention. A lack of hormones can reason blood strain to drop, muscle mass to weaken,

and ordinary fatigue to set in. Many who are sooner or later diagnosed with Addison's disorder regularly experience an Addisonian crisis first, which signals Doctors to adrenal insufficiency.

Risk elements for adrenal issues can fluctuate, but most instances are brought about by way of underlying autoimmune disorders. Other predetermining factors may include:

- Chronic diseases, such as tuberculosis
- Previous infections
- Surgeries that eliminated parts of adrenal glands
- Autoimmune diseases like Graves' disease, Lupus, or HIV
- Certain antifungal medicinal drugs

Symptoms of excessive stages of cortisone (Cushing's disease) include:

- Upper physique obesity, while palms and legs stay thinner. A common trait known as a Buffalo hump refers to a lump between the shoulders.

- Being worn out and confused.
- Developing high blood pressure and diabetes.
- Skin that bruises easily.
- Wide purplish streak marks on the stomach skin.

Symptoms of high tiers of aldosterone include:

- High blood pressure.
- Low potassium levels.
- Weakness.
- Pain and spasms in your muscles.

Symptoms of high ranges of male sex hormones are solely apparent in women or young boys earlier than puberty. These include:

- Growing facial hair and or balding.
- Developing acne.
- Having a deeper voice.
- Becoming more muscular.
- Developing an increased sex drive.
- Developing masculine qualities is known as virilization.

ADRENAL FATIGUE

If your body produces too many adrenal hormones, they accumulate in your waistline. Your physique gets stuck in "high alert" mode, and stress hormones are launched repeatedly because of the daily life hurdles; they can purpose adrenal exhaustion. It's one of the most recurring hormonal issues. Yet, many women and their doctors don't understand the warning signs of adrenal fatigue until it's too late. Learning to deal with stress responses is one of the most natural ways to stabilize hormones, reap safe weight, a healthful immune system, proper sleep, and stable moods.

During normal metabolic functions, the hormones tend to fluctuate for the human body to relax and respond accurately to the stimuli it receives. For example, much less cortisol will be secreted in the evening so that you may relax for sleep, and it ramps up in the early morning to supply strength for the day. But suppose you're stressed, either due to external circumstances or illness. In that case, the stage of corticosteroids can change dramatically and get caught in the "always-on" position from time to time.

If that happens, you may feel distressed even if there aren't any stressful triggers in your surroundings— and it can lead to adrenal insufficiency when the glands are unable to hold up with the demands placed on them.

Adrenal Fatigue and Weight Gain

One response could be weight fluctuation. Some people may experience weight loss, while others may see weight gain, with each effect occurring despite eating an identical quantity of calories.

The hypothalamic-pituitary-adrenal (HPA) axis gland is continuously working when you're stressed. This makes the adrenal glands secrete a lot of cortisol, which binds to fat cells. As a result, an enzyme- lipoprotein lipase is activated. Its job is to turn circulating triglycerides into free fatty acids, or FFA.3 The additional FFA you have, the less reactive insulin gets at its job of breaking down fat. The final result is weight gain!

Our adrenal glands govern our stress response with the aid of secreting hormones relative to our stress levels. Research states adrenal exhaustion in the latter arsenal extreme tiers of adrenal fatigue. It occurs when the adrenal glands, which produce cortisol in response to all types of stressors, are so exhausted that they can no longer produce the hormone in regular amounts to fight normal amounts of stress.

Whether the adrenal tumor inflicts Cushing's or subclinical Cushing's syndrome, one of the most common resultants of excessive cortisol is weight gain. Fat is also distributed in the cheeks. A hump can happen over the back of the neck due to fat distribution. It can also accumulate over the collar bones.

We already know that cortisol controls the stress response in the human body. But it's not just that; our body mechanisms alter to release such a hormone in response to stress. For instance, when you're distressed, your sugar levels are incredibly high, which aids the body in producing enough energy to overcome the stressful situation.

Sugar levels have a direct impact on your weight. We already know high cortisol increases insulin resistance, but what does that have to do with weight? Insulin doesn't just generate diseases in the human body, it can also trigger your stomach and make you feel more hungry than usual. When you continuously feel hungry, you rely more on sweet foods for fulfilling the inadequate energy because, let's face it, carbs are literally more delicious than anything you can think of. Hence, you experience weight gain. Adrenal fatigue becomes the concealed source that no one bats an eye to.

The Signs of Adrenal Fatigue

Following are the signs that indicate adrenal fatigue in the body.

▶ Low Energy

Low energy and fatigue are two of the most common reasons patients visit their doctors to find help. But despite being so prevalent, it can be challenging for medical professionals to conduct a diagnosis, as a varying number of diseases can cause tiredness and low energy. Among them, we find adrenal fatigue, which connects stress exposure to adrenal exhaustion as one of the causes of insufficient energy. Prolonged exposure to pressure and stress is thought to drain the adrenals, two small glands located on top of the kidneys that produce several hormones like cortisol. This adrenal depletion would produce fewer hormones than required by the body and cause various issues, including brain fog, depressive moods, but most importantly, low energy, and fatigue.

▶ Exhaustion

Unexplained exhaustion is another sign of adrenal fatigue closely related to low energy, in which case it's important to check with your doctor right away. They can diagnose your symptoms and run relevant tests to rule out other health problems. While medication can be crucial, you can do a few other things to help with exhaustion. For instance, eliminating cortisol-triggering foods like sugars, alcohol, and chocolate in addition to taking vitamin supplements and exercising daily with moderate intensity can do a lot for adrenal issues.

▶ Anxiety

Most people think of anxiety as just a mental health disorder that they need to get rid of to live a more peaceful life. When in actuality, anxiety is just the activation of a person's sympathetic nervous system, more commonly known as the fight or flight response, a system that's put in place to keep you safe from harm. Anxiety happens when your flight or fight response malfunctions. While the response itself is incredibly essential for our survival, its malfunction is what causes people distress. Anxiety and stress affect just about every gland in your body. While not all of the symptoms of anxiety arise from the endocrine system, many of them do. The endocrine system plays a huge role in releasing many of the hormones that create these symptoms. Reduced cortisol outputs tend to lead to physiological changes, which cause dire symptoms such as anxiety, depression, and lowered tolerance to stress. Anxiety caused by adrenal fatigue can badly impact your daily routine; therefore, it's best to consult a medical professional for this concern.

▶ Frequent Illness

Chronic diseases, such as asthma or arthritis, cause inflammation, which causes your body to respond hormonally. To combat inflammation, the adrenals produce and release cortisol and cortisone. The more severe the infection, the harder your adrenals must work. Chronic disease treatment can also be stressful on your body. Antibiotics and chemotherapy, for example, can put enormous strain on our endocrine system. And the fatigue caused by infections can lead to the development of habits that further weaken the adrenals, such as drinking more caffeine or using other stimulants.

▶ Difficulty Falling Asleep

Many of the symptoms of adrenal fatigue don't occur suddenly; they appear gradually and aren't that difficult to miss. Some of the first few signs of adrenal fatigue are constant tiredness, chronic fatigue, and muscle weakness, primarily due to the loss of sleep associated with it. In a healthy individual, cortisol production reaches its peak around 10 AM and declines to its lowest point before midnight, around 10 PM. These cortisol levels allow for a proper sleep and wake cycle. A disruption of cortisol production results in a disturbance of this routine cycle. The causes for this disruption can lie anywhere from relationship issues, intense work environments, poor diet, trauma-inducing situations, or anything that may result in chronic stress. The chronic stress from these high-pressure situations keeps your adrenals on constant alert, producing too much cortisol too often. This leads to insomnia, i.e., wakeful hours in the middle of the night and absent energy during the day.

▶ Frequent Urination

Polyuria, the medical term for your body producing more urine than normal, is a common condition that many people have and is often attributed to old age. Still, research has shown how adrenal fatigue can become a leading cause of this issue. Similarly, Sugar and salt cravings will develop as the adrenal gland and kidneys' glandular resources of fuel, minerals, and vitamins stored and available to the tissues are depleted, combined with skipping meals or overindulging in unopposed carbohydrates. This disrupts your blood sugar management system and hormone balance even more.

The cortex of the adrenal glands is in charge of producing aldosterone, a mineralocorticoid that works with the kidney to regulate fluid and mineral excretion. When the adrenal glands become exhausted, we produce less aldosterone and tend to excrete large amounts of important minerals in our urine. Individuals with depleted endocrine systems often report frequent urination, which is frequently attributed to age but may be caused by depleted adrenals.

This means that Adrenal Fatigue patients effectively lose the ability to balance mineral levels in their blood, such as sodium, potassium, and magnesium. As a result, we develop cravings for foods that will replace the sodium we have lost. If you suddenly crave salty snacks, you may be suffering from Adrenal Fatigue.

ADRENAL INSUFFICIENCY

Unlike adrenal fatigue, which can be difficult to diagnose and is questioned by various experts, adrenal insufficiency is a recognized disease that can be diagnosed. Adrenal insufficiency, which includes Addison's disease, is a disorder that happens when the adrenal glands inadequately produce certain hormones. Different types of adrenal insufficiency have varying causes, but the most common is the sudden cessation of consuming corticosteroids after taking them for a long period. The inability to increase cortisol levels with stress due to adrenal insufficiency can lead to what's known as an Addisonian crisis. An Addisonian crisis is a serious, life-threatening situation that causes low blood pressure and reduced sugar and potassium levels in the blood. This crisis requires immediate and expert medical care. There are mainly two forms of this condition, both of which are caused by damaged or problematic adrenal glands. Adrenal insufficiency is diagnosed through a blood test that determines if your cortisol levels are too low. If they are, then you require a hormone replacement.

HOW TO FIX ADRENAL FATIGUE AND LOWER CORTISOL LEVELS

Our bodies depend on a few key hormones that give us energy and keep our engines running smoothly. When these hormones aren't being produced as they should or insufficient amounts, they can leave us feeling tired, drained, and empty. The endocrine glands are responsible for secreting the hormones we need to survive and function every day, including cortisol and some sex hormones. So what can cause all these negative effects of adrenal fatigue?

Several adrenal disorders can affect the function of the adrenal glands. Genetic mutations can often be to blame, as can tumors, chronic infections, or medications. Problems with other glands, like the pituitary gland, can also be blamed as they help regulate and control the adrenal glands. Unfortunately, there is a large list of symptoms to expect with any case of adrenal fatigue.

If you want to know how to diagnose adrenal fatigue, a good place to start is to check how many of these common symptoms apply to you. Keep in mind that adrenal fatigue affects everyone differently, but there are specific effects that many people can experience. Cortisol, in particular, is a hormone affected by adrenal function.

Cortisol helps you respond to stress in normal, healthy ways. In addition, it maintains blood sugar levels, regulates the metabolism of fats, proteins, and carbohydrates, and controls the immune response.

The Three Stages of Cortisol Irregularity

Stage 1: Wired and exhausted

This stage is from extreme cortisol levels, particularly after dark, leading to restlessness, insulin opposition, and intestinal burden. People frequently feel energized without knowing the cause of having appropriate stimuli.

Stage 2: Stressed and exhausted

In this stage, many people revive early in the dawn and are powerless to retreat to sleep. Later in the epoch, agitation contributes, and they feel more awake. The cortisol levels rise, and they feel tired or stressed out by evening.

Stage 3: Burnout

This stage is from tiredness. You can feel exhausted despite getting a good night's sleep or even more hours than normal. It can affect your cortisol, thyroid hormone production, and DHEA.

Everyone knows that stress is a murderer of joy. All great afflictions like major diseases have stress contributing to their game. Whether it's coronary thrombosis (heart disease), tumor, or memory deficit, stress can cause it or affect your ability to overcome it. Most people living in societies are under plenty of stress due to their jobs, relationship issues, or other contributing stressors. And stress causes tiredness and fatigue. Overwhelming sensations are a welcome to unannounced stress in the human body; you can't appear to function right; your stress is consuming you. Another thing is that stress affects your physique. In addition, stress wears out the adrenal glands.

Fatigue is the ultimate root of all physical and mental problems. Your carcass demands extreme cortisol concentrations on the right occasions- especially during the day and depressed cortisol levels at added periods like at night. This keeps you fitted for routine adjustments so that you feel and function at your best.

There is a certain rhythm to cortisol levels, and any slight interference or disruption can broadly impact your life. Learning how to manage cortisol levels will prevent your hormones from working against you. But first, let's analyze this- what happens when cortisol levels are irregular or too high for the body to function normally?

Research shows that higher or even slightly moderate cortisol levels largely impact your bodily functions, which trip the metabolism into various health and energy consumption issues.

- Chronic affliction and diseases: Long-term raised cortisol levels grant an increased risk for severe cardiac disease, osteoporosis, myocardial infarction, type 2 diabetes, and other never-ending ailments.
- Difficulty in focusing: Also referred to as " brain fog," many people report trouble concentrating on anything and a lack of consciousness.
- Weight gain: Cortisol grants permission to increase hunger and signals the body to shift absorption to store fat.
- Lack of strength/trouble dormant(sleeping): It can obstruct sleep hormones that impact sleep conditions and time.
- Immune system troubles: Increased cortisol can hamper the order of the immune system, making it harder to fight contaminations and severe infections in the body.
- Cushing's syndrome: Sometimes, extreme cortisol levels can bring about this condition, a rare but weighty ailment.

▶ Get Plenty of Sleep

Prioritizing your sleep concedes the possibility of humble or controlling cortisol levels. Chronic sleep issues such as sleep apnea, restlessness, or shift working have been the root cause of rising cortisol levels. Outworking yourself is directly linked with poorer health outcomes. It's mandatory to get 8-10 hours a night. Your body recovers while you are sleeping.

Furthermore, insomnia is a sleep condition that refers to trouble dormant. It may be provoked by the entirety, containing stress and obstructive sleep apnea. This can influence the increased flowing of cortisol that influences your regular hormonal patterns and strength/energy levels. If you are a rotating shift employee, you do not have the position of great advantage over your sleep schedule, but there are a few things you can do to overcome it.

- Have a bedtime routine. Establishing a consistent bedtime routine can narrate your intellect and physique to start relaxing for the night.
- Go to bed and revive in the intervening time each day.

- Exercise earlier in the morning regularly. Exercising can automatically increase healthy sleep patterns.
- Limit hot beverages with caffeine intake. Try to reduce any caffeine intake about 6 hours before your time for bed.
- Avoid nicotine and alcohol intoxication. Both elements can influence sleep quality.
- Limit exposure to bright light each evening. Around 45–60 minutes before sleep, decrease the number of bright lights around you- especially in your bedroom. Instead of scrolling through your phone in bed, try reading a book or hearing to a podcast.
- Go to bed in a quiet range. Limit interruptions by utilizing acoustical noise, earplugs, and silencing all electronics.
- Take naps. If work cuts your sleep hours short, short naps can reduce lethargy and avert a required sleep.

Practicing good sleep hygiene can help hold cortisol levels in a sane beat. The above-listed remedies are direct strategies for good sleep.

▶ Exercise, but Not Excessively

Depending on the exercise force, it can increase or decrease cortisol- light cardio and weight training are best. Consistent high-intensity training increases cortisol levels. Try yoga; it relaxes your mind and body, lowering cortisol levels. Intense exercise increases cortisol quickly but will decrease it hours later. This temporary increase helps coordinate the development of the physique to meet the challenge. Additionally, the proportion of the cortisol response lessens accompanying routine preparation.

Regular exercise has been proved in abundant studies to help enhance sleep conditions, humble stress, and upgrade overall health, which can help lower cortisol gradually but surely. Interestingly, routine exercise has further shown to execute higher resilience to severe stress and may lower the risk of acquiring any negative health affect associated with stress or excessive cortisol. In addition, overplaying it can have the opposite effect. Therefore, rely on about 140–200 minutes of exercise for the entire week and allow yourself to rest between workouts. Exercising can help you better control stress and promote the best condition, which can help lower cortisol levels.

▶ Learn to Acknowledge Stress

Paying attention to anxious thoughts will help you defeat them easily. Stress reduction is a game plan that includes suitable, more self-consciousness of stress-provoking concepts, recognizing and accepting them without judgment or fighting, and admitting yourself the strength to process your thoughts. Training yourself to be informed about your recurring negative thoughts, effect on respiratory patterns, cardiac rhythms, and different signs of tension help you admit stress when it starts.

By fixating on knowledge of your mental and material state, you can enhance an objective spectator of your difficult thoughts rather than allowing them to become a casualty for you. Recognizing difficult thoughts will help you form a plan on how to tackle them. Therefore, try practicing a better conscious response to stressors in your routine for better stress administration and reduced cortisol levels.

Practicing mental care can help you label tense concepts and manage your thoughts accurately. Mindfulness-based practices are the only addition to your life that will help you defeat stress and lower cortisol levels.

▶ Breathe

Breathing is a straightforward technique for stress decline that may be unspecified secondhand areas. Like mindfulness practice, regulated breathing helps excite the parasympathetic central nervous system, known as the "rest and digest" scheme, which helps lower cortisol levels. Studies have proved decreases in cortisol in participants that included deep breathing into their grooves. This type of practice is common in mental relief practices in addition to yoga and Tai chi, where skill is of decisive importance.

Multiple studies validate that these practices can help lower cortisol and accomplish reduced stress. Deep breathing activates the parasympathetic nervous system, freeing up mental energy, and lowering cortisol levels. Any form of meditation can be used as an alternative because almost all meditative patterns include deep breathing as a primary element.

▶ Have Fun

Another habit of keeping cortisol low is by having fun and enjoying life. Laughing advances the release of endorphins and suppresses stress hormones like cortisol. It further accompanies better mood, diminished stress and pain, lowers heart rate, and boosts the immune system. Interestingly, real and compulsory amusement can lead to lower levels of stress. Laughing — advances deliberate rounds of amusement — has been proved to lower cortisol levels, humble stress, and increase energy levels by improving mood. Developing avocations can further advance feelings of wellness, which can lower cortisol. Tending to your happiness can help maintain cortisol levels. If you're impression emphasized, try listening to pleasant sounds or harmonized music.

▶ Be Yourself

Feelings of shame, blame, or defeat can lead to a bad attitude and raised cortisol. For a few blame causes, repairing the source will mean making a change in your history. For additional causes, knowledge to excuse and accept yourself and help you proceed and enhance your sense of prosperity. Developing a habit of forgiveness is essential in relationships. Resolving guilt executes feelings of vindication and lowers cortisol levels. It involves changing practices, making merciful choices, or learning to excuse yourself.

If you grant yourself religion, developing your conviction can further help upgrade cortisol levels. Studies show that people with spiritual faith and contentment are usually far happier than those with low to no faith. Belief is a powerful force that occupies the mind and reduces any feelings of fear or stress.

Suppose you exclude yourself from these acts of faith and religion. In that case, being humble in general and having an empathic approach to all human beings around you- operating acts of generosity may be the solution to lowering your cortisol levels, encompassing adrenal fatigue, and maintaining a healthy lifestyle.

▶ Eat a Healthy Diet

Nutrition can influence cortisol for the better or worse. Eat the right food for your body. For instance,

- Be cautious of food sensitivities which can add extra stress on your system, bloating, and fatigue.
- Eat in at regular intervals, about the same time every day. It helps stabilize blood sugars and energy levels.
- Minimize sugar intake. Beware of hidden sugars, i.e. dextrose, maltose, and agave syrup.
- Eat any starchy carbohydrates earlier in the day when cortisol levels are raised.
- Minimal or no caffeine intake. Caffeine

increases adrenal hormones, causing
adrenaline to increase by 32% and
noradrenaline by 14%. Suppose you have a
caffeine sensitivity, i.e. shaking, heart
palpitations, trouble speaking, anxiety, you
may want to cut out caffeine.

- Don't completely cut out carbs. Too low intake
  can increase cortisol levels by 18% and reduce
  the thyroid T3 hormone.

While all types of food can be savored to a degree, being attentive to the cooking you nibble on may lessen manifestations of stress and help you better control your cortisol levels. Research has proved a strong connection between a healthy gut microbiome — all the bacteria filling a place in your gut — and improved physical and mental fitness. Therefore, absorbing snacks to support a healthy gut can help lower stress and worry and develop your overall energy.

Other foods that are beneficial for directing cortisol involve,

- Dark chocolate: Studies show that our brain
  interprets the sensations of eating chocolate

same as the feeling of falling in love- it makes us happy and relieved. Dark chocolate contains many flavonoids, which have proven to buffer stress responsiveness to stimuli in the adrenal glands, resulting in lower cortisol release.

- Whole grains: Unlike other grains, whole grains are rich in polyphenols and texture, which can support stress levels and gut energy.
- Legumes and lentils: They're extreme in texture that supports a healthy gut while directing glucose levels.
- Fruits and Vegetables: Whole fruits and salads hold a plethora of antioxidants and polyphenolic compounds that fight container-damaging free radicals.
- Green tea: Green tea holds a famous appeasing compound, L-theanine, which happens to be connected to decreased stress and raised alertness.
- Probiotics and prebiotics: Probiotics are companionable, cooperative microorganisms found in yogurt, sauerkraut, and kimchi. Prebiotics, to a degree dissolved texture, support food for these microorganisms. Both

probiotics and prebiotics are connected to a
better gut microbiome and increased energy.

- Healthy fats: A diet high in unsaturated fat is
  full of energy. In particular, end-3 oily acids
  are best for weakening stress.

- Water: Dehydration causes a transient
  increase in cortisol levels, making it even more
  important to drink water throughout the
  whole day.

CHAPTER 3
STEP 3: GET TO KNOW YOUR SUPERFOODS

NUTRITION AND WEIGHT LOSS

Whether you've been attempting to lose weight for a few weeks or a few years, it's inevitable to get annoyed by the notion over time. Many people feel let down by the dietary plans they've been following for a significant period and feel that something's still missing. As someone suffering from the absurdity of weight gain, you'd know that little to no progress doesn't matter when tons of emerging inconveniences such as turbulent hunger seem to never leave your side whether or not you choose to go on a diet. The result is a constant war with the weighing scale. Maintaining a healthy weight is critical for looking fit, feeling fit, and even dwelling in a wholesome lifestyle.

Losing bodyweight or retaining a consistent body weight consists of benefits like reduced LDL cholesterol and blood sugar levels, lower blood pressure, less stress on bones and joints, and reduced risk of heart diseases. Nutrition is the single most exclusive weight loss management and fitness maintenance component. The best of us have a distinct love for food, and fortunately, in our world, we have no shortage of choices. But, the only question that remains is what does one mean by proper nutrition?

Good nutrition denotes consuming ingredients to get the nutrients essential for providing energy to your body. Nutrients are the chemical compounds your body needs, such as macronutrients like protein, carbohydrates, and fat, and micronutrients, like nutritional vitamins and minerals. Good nutrition is a proper plan instigated to avoid packaged or processed foods as much as possible. These foods have excessive quantities of sodium and a long list of ingredients that are unfamiliar to our digestive systems. When you consume so much of something that your body takes longer to adjust to, it disrupts your digestive patterns- allowing your body to grow more fat instead of decomposing the food to derive energy.

A healthy diet also proposes monitoring any introduced sugar forms in your food and limiting your sugar intake. Once your body's strength requirements are fulfilled, all the extra energy is stored as fat. Some of the remaining food portions are stored as glycogen inside your muscles for strength, but the majority is accumulated as fat at different body portions. So ingesting greater energy than you burn will result in weight gain, like less energy than you require will result in unhealthy weight loss.

Most people misunderstand fat consumption as something entirely unhealthy and a factor to be eliminated from its core. However, when our bodies have consumed enough energy for the day and are unable to utilize the extra energy or strength existing because of digested food, we come geared up with an outstanding energy storage device referred to as fat. Some fats are essential for keeping us healthy, so no one should be striving for zero percent fat. However, most of us retain a few greater layers than we need.

Most of us are perplexed by multiple questions, how much diet do I need for a better shape? How many meals do I skip until I look like I want? Is the sole vegetable diet the only way to a healthy metabolism? Will my hormones function normally if I skip all the protein from my regular food intake? Can big changes affect our previous horrific habits and let us have a body that will make anybody flip their heads toward us? Too many questions – and a big pile of data that the media, nutritionists, and health lovers confuse us with doesn't help much.

Good nutrition can assist you in shedding excess pounds — barring meal cravings or feeling hungry! This is because wholesome ingredients are packed with nutrients, not like processed foods, which are usually loaded with fat, sugar, and salt. Nutritional deficiencies are what cause cravings for quick-energy-fix meals like candy and chips. Without them, you give in to your unhealthy cravings. So, why do human beings resist diets?

One of the motives many humans drawback at the phrase "diet" is the thinking about all the times they'll be feeling hungry and grumpy, skipping their favorite meals, and cutting down on the extra snacks that give them fuel to battle the struggles of the rest of the day. Maybe it's because people, despite their desire to change something in their health routine, feel it's tougher to choose when it comes to such steps. They depart those few extra kilos to dangle around as they aren't positive, which is the right way to make them healthy again without endangering their health.

Food is the groundwork for a healthy lifestyle and any form of adjustments in our body. The tremendous impact is constantly noticeable when we eat yummy foods and take beneficial nutrients. Nutrition does not simply contain the meals you devour in a day. It additionally has a lot to do with what you drink. The only high-quality fluid you need to consume regularly is water. It is calorie-free, and it is essential for all life functions. The reality is that there is no miracle weight-loss shake despite what the internet must say.

All healthy weight loss comes from a healthy diet or burning extra power from food than you take in. Sometimes we aren't even aware of how many distinct kinds of meals our body needs to get a proper dose of all the required nutrients. Instead, we often have a habit of relying on a single type of component because it might also be simpler for us to prepare it than to come up with new ideas. Hence for your convenience, here are 33 healthy superfoods you can use as an alternative to processed snacks.

33 SUPERFOODS FOR WEIGHT LOSS SUCCESS

Carbohydrates

1. Tomatoes – are low in calories, low in fat, and rich in fiber. It has a fat-burning compound called 9-oxo-ODA. Contains antioxidants that help keep off illness and disease.

2. Grapefruit – activates fat-burning hormones and suppresses appetite.

3. Beetroot – low in calories, high in fiber, and magnesium. Contains phytonutrients that reduce inflammation.

4. Hot peppers - contain capsaicin, which helps turn food into energy and aids in burning abdominal fat.

5. Apples – High in pectin; binding to water limits the amount of fat your cells can absorb. High in fiber – it keeps you full longer.

6. Pears – also contain pectin (same benefits as apples).

7. Cantaloupe – Contains the fat-burning compound beta-carotene.

8. Bananas – Contains soluble fiber, which helps slow digestion and keeps you full longer.

9. Blueberries – Contains high amounts of

polyphenol oxidants that burn fat and prevent fat from forming.

10. Strawberries – contain soluble fiber that slows the stomach's emptying rate and gives the feeling of satiety longer.

11. Oranges – Boosts vitamin C, are low in calories, and fiber helps regulate blood sugar.

12. Sweet potato – digested slowly, contains nutrients that lower blood sugar and insulin resistance. Helps the digestive system work properly.

13. Asparagus – natural diuretic. Helps expel toxins and other waste from the body. Aids in digestion – feeds the guts good bacteria, and is high in vitamins and minerals.

14. Mushrooms – Aids in weight loss. Contains no fat or sugar.

15. Broccoli – Low in calories and helps you feel full, high in nutrients and fiber.

16. Spinach – High in fiber, low in calories.

17. Ginger – contains antioxidants that help control damage from free radicals and contain anti-inflammatory agents.

18. Oats – High in fiber- slows digestion and aids in the feeling of satiety, and boosts metabolism.

19. Beans – High in fiber, keeps you full longer, slows down digestion.

20. Lentils – High in protein and a good fiber source, they keep you satisfied between meals.

21. Chia Seeds – contain high amounts of fiber and antioxidants. High in Omega-3 fatty acids and amino acids.

Proteins

22. Quinoa – is a complete protein (contains the complete chain of amino acids necessary for muscle building and fat loss)

23. Eggs – high in lean protein and healthy fat with good cholesterol.

24. Salmon – excellent quality protein, healthy fat, high in nutrients that help burn fat, build muscle, and aid in weight loss by blocking fat storage.

25. Greek yogurt – lots of protein, little sugar.

Fats

26. Nuts – high in healthy calories – keeps you full. Contain nutrients that promote weight loss.

27. Pine nuts – contain a phytonutrient that helps suppress appetite.

28. Flax seeds - high in vitamins and minerals and are a good source of omega-3 and fiber. Lowers bad cholesterol. Boosts metabolism.

29. Avocados - contain vitamin B (mood boosters) and lower stress levels. Prevents body fat distribution around the stomach.

30. Coconut oil – easily digested fat. Converts directly into energy – not stored as fat. Stimulates metabolism.

31. Extra virgin olive oil – anti-inflammatory; contains nutrients that benefit fat loss.

Beverages

32. Green tea – contains the antioxidant ECGC, which triggers the release of fat from cells, increasing your liver's ability to turn fat into energy. It speeds up metabolism.

33. Apple Cider Vinegar (raw) – Acidic foods

increase your metabolism and lead to weight loss. Enzymes in apple cider vinegar help digest food and regulate blood sugar.

7 FOODS TO AVOID

You may think eating habits have nothing to do with diet, but it does. Many people suffering from weight gain embark on the exhausting journey of regular diet and exercise only to find out they've been doing it all wrong. Isn't it confusing when you've been following each step accurately of a popular diet on the internet or a suggestion from a fitness-passionate friend? However, it goes to waste in the end because there's no apparent change in your weight, and besides, you feel incredibly hungry no matter how many healthy foods/snacks you consume. So, where does it all go wrong?

While it's not important to avoid every food when it comes to diet, there are certain red flags you must completely avoid if you want a healthier lifestyle, let alone a diet. There isn't such a long list of compulsories, but a summary of some edibles our palettes desire more than our bodies' metabolisms.

1. Baked foods – ie. Cookies, pastries, and other desserts. High in sugar and trans fats. Most people naturally have a sweet tooth which means they are drawn to almost anything sweet, and that's great unless your body has a negative reaction to every second piece of candy you consume. Desserts have the core ingredient you need to limit if you want a healthier lifestyle- sugar. It's important to find healthy dessert alternatives for accurate weight loss provisions.

2. White pasta and bread – refined wheat flour are high in calories and low in fiber, breaking down a lot faster and causing blood sugar spikes. It also lacks protein and other nutrients.

3. White rice – Minimal fiber and protein. Fiber and protein are the two things you want your body to consume for weight loss to be healthy. Weight losing diets mainly comprise of foods that starve you to your bones until the retrograde to a healthy body is impossible.

4. Most energy and granola bars – tend to be high in sugar. A better option is to make a healthy version at home, like a combination of Greek yogurt and any type of berries.

5. Processed meat – meaning manufacturers

have either smoked, dried, fermented, canned, or processed and preserved. Tend to be high in salt and low in nutrients. It is classified as a carcinogen. Buy freshly cut meat for any homemade meal. Please don't cut down on protein; find a healthy way to ingest it.

6. French fries and potato chips – are typically cooked in a deep fryer adding unhealthy fat and calories. A lack of protein and fiber reduces the amount of time you will feel satisfied. A healthy diet consists of foods that give you energy for the rest of the day and minimize the body's need to eat additional snacks.

7. Alcohol - Sugary and calorie-dense. No nutritional value. Keeps fat on the midsection. It is also dangerous to health in every way and form. Hence, cutting down alcoholic consumption from your lifestyle progresses toward a healthy body and diet.

VITAMINS THAT ASSIST IN BALANCING HORMONES

Our first assumption, when our moods remotely fluctuate, is that our brain is responsible for the change. While that's not entirely incorrect, there are certain times distinct changes in our bodies are solely respon-sible for our disposition adaptations. Our hormones play a vital role in determining our moods, and these hormones are not released from the brain but from the endocrine system interconnected and spread within the human body. For instance, as mentioned a couple of times earlier, the hormone cortisol is responsible for stressor signals and responses within our body. When-ever you feel the slightest amount of stress, cortisol is in action.

Returning to the matter at hand, vitamins affect certain aspects of our lifestyles, including hormones that play a major role in balancing our lifestyles. Hormones are responsible for regulating more than enough functions in our body. Any slight change in vitamin consumption, such as a deficiency, will drastically affect the entire sequence of those regulations. Why is it important for weight loss? Like everything else mentioned up until now, weight loss is related to the most minor elements present in our body that go unnoticed. That's why most weight loss routines, diets, and exercises fail to prosper. There are many ways you can attain an unhealthy weight loss that impacts your health and leaves you, victim, to certain diseases that take a lifetime to unravel. However, there are just a handful of provisions to pursue when it comes to attaining good health and managing a prolonged ideal lifestyle.

Suppose you've recently come across a case of hormonal imbalance in your body. In that case, you must start by idealizing the number of vitamin deficiencies you may be fostering, as a lack of vitamins in the body is a major cause of imbalanced hormones. For instance, many people with vitamin D deficiencies fall victim to numerous diseases and have unexplained physical and mental changes that challenge multiple aspects of their lives. To conclude, here are vitamins essential for hormonal balance that you must include in your weight loss and diet routine for a healthy lifestyle.

- Omega 3 - A higher intake of omega3 can lower insulin resistance.
- Vitamin C – Aids in reducing adrenalin and cortisol levels.
- Vitamin B5, B6, and B12 – are needed for a properly functioning metabolism. B vitamins are responsible for metabolizing carbs, proteins, and fats and using the energy in food.
- Vitamin D – helps reduce the feeling of depression.

- Iron – helps the body make energy from nutrients. Carries oxygen throughout the body and helps burn fat.
- Ashwagandha – Helps reduce cortisol levels. Reduces depression and anxiety. Reduces blood sugar levels and inflammation. Improves sleep.
- Gymnema Sylvestre (Gurmar) – helps lower blood sugar levels and reduce cravings.
- Magnesium – is important for energy production. Assists in controlling blood pressure and blood sugar levels, keeping bones strong, and the nervous system functioning smoothly.

FOODS THAT IMPROVE YOUR MOOD

How many times have you found yourself in a situation when you're undeniably stressed or having a generally bad day, and your mind ultimately diverts to the thought of your favorite food or a general craving? Now you know food and mood go hand-in-hand. Cravings are just some innate humane feelings; they are literal signals from your mind that your body needs a specific type of food at that moment to recover from mental or physical exhaustion.

Sometimes most feelings or reactions are considered innate, but a little in-depth research leads you to discover the depths of your creation and how everything has a different logic behind it. Reverting to the point, wouldn't any mere craving impact your diet? Can a craving have an equivalent exchange- something that delivers the same satisfactory sensation to your taste-buds and doesn't leave any room for other hunger or starvation?

It is easily observable that whenever someone is going through a loss or a distressing situation, they automatically avert their attention to food and consume whatever they can until they've gained those extra pounds they weren't targeting. Food contains carbohydrates and protein that play an important part in creating and transmitting serotonin throughout the human body. Serotonin is a hormone that plays a vital role in improving your mood. The food you consume contains protein that is responsible for creating serotonin, and carbohydrates carry it from one place to another inside your body.

Hence, if you're looking for something to improve your mood, it may just be your favorite food. In addition, dietary changes affect your mental health. There are chronic mental disorders like depression and anxiety that limit your intake of food very naturally and diminish any feelings of hunger you may be feeling. Research suggests that dietary changes may also positively impact these mental health disorders.

While a momentary food intake can improve your mood, it can also impact your health and weight gain. These distinct dietary changes like irregular food consumption, especially foods that leave the fat in the midsection and don't benefit your body, can damage your physique. Studies show that a good dietary plan is eating well in the morning and slowly reducing the amount of food you consume throughout the day-towards the night. While it's mandatory to eat three times a day, you must preview what you're consuming and the amount of pressure you put your digestive system under. Comfort foods- the type of foods you intake during cravings- have a vast effect on your appetite, resulting in weight gain. But a weight loss routine doesn't mean entirely cutting down on comfort foods and never giving in to your cravings. Healthy weight-loss diets are all about food consumption in the right amounts at the right time and avoiding foods your body doesn't have the energy to digest or accept for the time being. Following that, some healthy foods play an essential part in improving your mood.

- Salmon - Omega 3 fatty acids help reduce anxiety.
- Green tea – lowers depressive symptoms.
- Blueberries – contain an antioxidant called flavonoids, which help regulate mood, improve memory, and protect your brain from aging.
- Green leafy vegetables – contain magnesium which aids in reducing anxiety.
- Dark chocolate – lowers cortisol levels.

ADDITIONAL BENEFITS OF GOOD NUTRITION

▶ Fuel to Function Everyday Activities

Every single act carried out by using your body – no count number of how small or mundane the venture may appear – requires energy. Proteins, fat, and carbohydrates all make contributions to the total power pool of the body. But for the body to be in a position to use and conserve this energy, it additionally wishes for positive nutritional vitamins and minerals, which can be acquired from meals and, to a lesser extent, supplements.

A weight loss program deficient in ingredients that grant energy and the critical vitamins and minerals to make this power available can lead to serious fitness problems, not to communicate starvation. By making sure suited energy, vitamin and mineral intake via the skill of the meals you eat, you may grant your body the necessary fuel to do all the duties required to keep life. Tasks like production and maintenance of the body tissues, nerve activity, muscle effort, and heat manufacturing to preserve body temperature require energy to prosper. The energy we get from food. But not all kinds of food.

▶ Nutrition for Precise Cell Functions

Our bodies function by using the capability of a highly complex set of structures that work in perfect synch to make existence possible. For instance, all these systems, the cardiovascular, reproductive, and respiratory systems, can be broken down into cell stages where hormones, enzymes, and neurotransmitters are continuously interacting via complicated methods to make your body function.

These processes are all made feasible through the vitamins we ingest each day. While the physique itself can produce specific vitamins, we want to get many others via the food we eat. An eating regimen deficient in vital vitamins will quickly lead to multiple chronic diseases.

By eating ingredients from various exclusive sources —
each animal-based and plant-based — you will furnish
your organs with the quintessential vitamins cells need
to have to function.

▶ Growth and Tissue Repair

Do you know how when a construction worker takes
over a project, they want the best possible materials for
renovation or construction of the particular site? Well,
our bodies function in a very similar manner. Good
nutrition ensures growth (during childhood and pregnancy), recovery, and muscle mass maintenance and
build-up. For these critical approaches to take place,
the body wants energy. The energy you can give it
through food. Sure some nutritional vitamins and
minerals fill up the space for energy. However, our body
needs protein on an everyday basis which we can only
consume through proper nutrition.

You can easily obtain protein from multiple resources,
particularly from animal products such as meat, eggs,
and milk. It also resources 17 kilojoules of power per
gram. Whey protein has been proven to have the most
advantageous absorption properties, which means your
physique can absorb and use the protein more effectively than different protein sources. Although the

western eating regimen generally incorporates ample protein, vegetarians can also be getting too little of this integral nutrient.

If you are a vegetarian, you must make a factor such as protein-rich meals in your diet. The benefit is that, should you suffer an injury, your body will be equipped and able to restore the broken tissue. You will also be capable of maintaining your muscle mass and making it bigger when you exercise. Magnesium, glucosamine, calcium, and vitamin D are imperative for bone and muscle increase and repair, so consider taking dietary supplements containing these elements if you are concerned your weight-reduction plan might also be deficient.

▶ Reinforcing the Immune System

You can allow your body to fight sickness extra efficaciously with the ingredients you eat. You, in all likelihood, already comprehend that vitamin C in oranges helps to ward off infection. This diet boosts immunity by employing growing the production of B- and T-cells and different white blood cells, along with those that break foreign microorganisms.

Similarly, other foods and vitamins can play an immune-boosting role. The key is to optimize your consumption of plant-based foods, such as fruit, vegetables, grains, nuts, and legumes. Including more omega-3 fatty acids in your food plan by ingesting extra fish while cutting down on your saturated fat consumption is also important.

Probiotics (microbial meals or dietary supplements that can re-establish the intestinal plant life in your gastrointestinal tract) also seem to kick the immune system up to your probiotic consumption by ingesting more low-fat or fat-free yogurt made with stay AB cultures.

▶ Preventing Continual Illnesses – A Secure Lifestyle

Good nutrition can be used as a device to combat persistent illnesses of lifestyle. Here, one of the essential steps is to obtain and keep a healthy weight by following an energy-controlled diet. It is a popular truth that obesity and overweight can lead to continual diseases, like diabetes type 2, coronary heart disease, hypertension, osteoarthritis, and some cancers.

Start by way of cutting out the saturated fats and introducing sugars. Also, make a point of consisting of extra plant-based meals in your diet. Plant-based meals usually have a lower fat content, are rich in fiber, and are additionally excellent sources of phytochemicals. More and more significant research points to the shielding houses of these supplies that manifest naturally in plants.

Phytochemicals appear to be of specific use in preventing cancer and coronary heart sickness by the procedure of neutralizing free radicals. In addition, they thwart enzymes that spark off cancer-causing sellers in the body.

▶ Maintaining Proper Mental Health

Diet can play a vital function in fighting off the blues. In preventing despair and temper swings, the primary principle is to devour a balanced weight-reduction plan that incorporates ingredients from all the excellent food sources. Here are a few essentials to put things in perspective.

- Never skip your fruit and vegetables. No matter what kind.
- Add unprocessed grains and cereals to your diet.
- Consume lean meat and eggs in the right amount.
- Don't completely avoid milk and dairy

products unless you have a negative reaction to them.

- Legumes, nuts, polyunsaturated or monounsaturated margarine, and oils are essential parts of a good diet.
- Also, make a point of inclusion for foods like fatty fish, salmon, and tuna in your diet. People who have an omega-3 deficiency are extra prone to depression than those who eat ample quantities.
- There is proof to endorse that an exact diet, and sufficient consumption of the omega-3s, can additionally assist in stopping Alzheimer's sickness in later life.

▶ Healthy Teeth and Bones

A nutritious weight-reduction plan also ensures the fitness of your enamel and bones. A balanced, calcium-rich diet – especially for the duration of your childhood, teen, and early adult years – has the benefit that it will make certain enough top bone mass throughout life. Calcium intake at required tiers will greatly help stop osteoporosis in later life.

A glass of milk includes around 300mg worth of calcium which makes it a required amount of calcium from one diet alone, so if you are worried about growing your calcium intake, you can try some calcium supplements. Adequate vitamin D3 stages help make sure your body can take in any calcium you consume - your each day consumption of Vitamin D3 is commonly acquired utilizing direct sunshine on the skin, but getting sufficient solar during winter months can be challenging, so a diet D supplement may additionally be beneficial to ensure bone strength.

You can also make certain your teeth' fitness by way of keeping a close eye on what you eat. Here's how you can do that.

- Try edibles such as cheese, nuts, popcorn, and vegetables if you want to snack on some food.
- Limit your between-meal consumption.
- Limit fermentable carbohydrates, like sugary drinks, from your life.
- Restrict any sugary treats.
- Ensure to consume a glass of water with every meal.

CHAPTER 4
STEP 4: UNDERSTAND NUTRIENT TIMING

THE ROLE OF MACRONUTRIENTS

The whole episode of weight loss unravels into whatever you're consuming at the end of the day. No matter how many websites influence you, weight loss is directly related to devouring your nutrients. Nutrients highly influence our hormones. If our bodies do not get proper nutrition, they will most likely submit to all the extra fat accumulation. What makes it so hard to lose weight?

The primary cause preventing successful weight loss is even though most people accurately follow a diet, their bodies do not get enough time to process all the energy. Macronutrients are essential components for the biological processes, also known as metabolisms occurring inside our bodies. They help the human body absorb and process mandatory vitamins for accurate hormonal function and balance. Hence, one way or another, minor aspects of your food, such as the consumption of macronutrients, are essential for the body- and ultimately for health and fitness.

Even though to lose weight, you have to maintain a lower calorie count; it's essential to preview how much energy does whatever you're eating giving you. Also, if the nutrients are enough to keep your body fit and healthy, they leave no additional room for hunger. What most people miss when trying to lose weight is idealizing and acknowledging the quality of their calories. The most challenging part of losing weight is when you're looking at yourself in the mirror after an intense workout for weeks and undernourished or hollow dieting, only to discover the extra fat that made you self-conscious and insecure and motivated you to lose weight in the first place. Hence, if you must lose those couple of extra pounds, you might as well accomplish it in the healthiest way possible.

Given that, macronutrients are smaller portions of your food if you put it more straightforwardly. Each type of food contains different enzymes and compounds. Similarly, macronutrients comprise carbohydrates, fats, and protein. Many people cut carbohydrates entirely out of their lives when they pursue a diet to become the most unhealthy and weak version of themselves. They don't realize the importance of macronutrients and don't bother investigating the nutrients in their weight loss diets. Anything you eat in a routine becomes a diet for your body. Your body slowly becomes accustomed to consuming the same amount of food at the same time; hence, entirely altering its course of the procession may be a little hectic at first.

You might have heard people telling you how they lost all this weight by completing cutting down carbs from their lives. But what you don't know is how it affects their mood. Carbohydrates play an essential role in supporting the functions of your brain throughout the day. Hence, completely removing them from your diet may have a drastic impact on your brain- it may even alter your mood from time to time and eventually cause a much worse hormonal imbalance. Similarly, protein is essential to give your bone and muscles strength, so they give you enough energy to carry out the day. Hence, removing something like that from your diet will make you disabled one way or another. You may even accomplish weight loss, but you'll feel starved all the time, unhappy and distressed without any stressful stimuli in the environment, and even with the perfect diet and exercise, your body won't have enough energy to do the simplest of things. We do all this to get rid of fat, but what are we missing?

Each unit of fat contains almost nine calories; anyone can quickly see how that can be alarming. But despite that, our body needs fat consumption as it's the primary component of giving us energy. And remember, a healthy amount of fat consumed helps burn extra fat and keeps you fit. On the contrary, a low fat intake can impact your entire wellbeing because it suppresses metabolic activities and slows hormone functions, resulting in hormonal imbalance and obesity. The macro ratio for fat loss is 40-50% protein, 30-40% fat, and 10-30% carbohydrate. That is because,

- Protein is vital when it comes to weight loss. It helps keep you full longer, boosts metabolism, and aids in regulating hormones. A higher protein intake increases the satiety hormone levels and reduces the levels of ghrelin (hunger hormone), therefore decreasing caloric intake. A higher protein diet leads to reduced cravings. Eating more protein will help keep muscle mass in your body and prevent your metabolism from slowing down; you will burn belly fat, not muscle. Although meat sources are what most people go to when consuming a protein source, a vegetarian and vegan diet can be just as effective when eating a healthy balanced diet.

- Carbohydrates break down into sugar or glucose, which your body uses as fuel. It's essential to understand the difference between good and bad carbohydrates when wanting to lose weight. Focus on carbs that contain fiber; they break down slower, so there is a lower spike in blood sugar levels. Some carbohydrates offer little nutritional value, causing your blood sugars to rise. You must consume healthy carbohydrates to lose weight.

- Fats are essential for good health and a staple in the human diet. Saturated fats are high in calories helping us stay full longer. They help digest protein and carbs.

It is one of the many reasons now specialists itch the whole idea of counting your calories because it's not essential. What's important is to measure the quality of each calorie intake, and macronutrients help you with that. Because a monitored intake of healthy carbs, lean protein, and wholegrain foods can balance your hormones and simultaneously give you a calorie deficit diet. To conclude, the latest studies on achieving hormonal balance to acquire a healthy weight loss propose that anyone can achieve a calorie deficit diet by monitoring the intake of macronutrients.

HEALTHY EATING HABITS

What does it mean by healthy eating habits mean? Does it mean that you get a list of the foods you must eat throughout the day repeatedly without any comprehension of what not to feel afterward? How many times have you eaten during the day and still felt like you had an empty stomach an hour later? Doesn't it feel strange when you go on a new diet, and the first thing you feel after a "healthy" meal is hunger and starvation- like something's still missing? And as before, the mind collapses into a labyrinth of endless questions of whether or not this is the proper diet for you? Or you should browse through the internet to find other relevant dietary plans that may work for you. And then, a month or two later, you've given up on a diet and are on an endless spree of insecurity and self-consciousness that slowly makes you give up.

So, where does it all go wrong? Even though specialists all over the web and television tell you what to eat and what not to eat, what they exclude from that list is the exhausting feeling of hunger that doesn't leave you until you've either given up on a diet or become weak rather than fit. Creating a healthy eating habit is all about monitoring the food intake and how much energy it's going to give you, how much time your body takes to absorb it (when you start feeling hungry again) and how healthy you'll look and feel.

Your goal isn't to become skinny but healthy. The well-known and conventional phrase "an apple a day will keep the doctor away" is there for a reason. You must never skip fruits or vegetables from your diet. Generally, adding fruits and vegetables to your diet can reduce the risk of any health problems, especially Type II diabetes. Not to mention, you'll be in a better mood constantly. When you're feeling great, the atmosphere is uplifted, and you're more prepared to battle any challenges that come your way. When we eat a healthful diet, our brain activity is regulated, and we're able to make sound decisions. Hence, a good lifestyle is just some healthy eating habits away from you.

Here are some pointers for what eating habits to adopt for weight loss.

1. Eat high protein food at every meal—30-40grams of protein.
2. Eat vegetables with each meal—two servings of vegetables.
3. Eat healthy fats daily.
4. Eat the majority of carbohydrates in the morning or after exercise.
5. Eat slowly.
6. Stop eating when you feel 80% full.
7. Drink lots of water.

Alarms During Diets

- Immediately after eating, you might feel a little bit hungry because it takes about 15-20 minutes to get the sense that you are no longer hungry.
- 1 hour after eating, you should still feel full and have no desire to eat.
- 2 hours after eating, you should start to feel a little bit hungry but still have no desire to eat a meal.
- 3 hours after eating, you should feel hungry for

a meal but not to the point of feeling like you are starving.

- 4 hours after eating, you should feel like you are starving. Do not let your body get to this point.

NUTRIENT TIMING - WHEN SHOULD I EAT?

Now that you know you must monitor your food intake, especially the macronutrients, it's only fair to let you in on the secrets of nutrient timing. Many fitness gurus are ready to answer queries on what to eat, but no one ever pays attention to when you should eat it.

The human body requires a specific type of food at different intervals of the day. On the road to fitness, it's our responsibility to take care of our body and learn how to cherish it. The primary aspect of monitoring nutrient timing is to work on the intake of carbohydrates. Our body takes a distinct amount of time to absorb each type of carbohydrate. That is because it controls the insulin response of the body. Insulin is mandatory for the human body because it gives us multiple muscle growth-related benefits. There's a specific interval of the day where if you take a large number of carbohydrates, it helps you control the insulin ratio and, in turn, enhances the functioning capacity of your body.

We consume refined carbohydrates, which contain compounds that trigger cholesterol levels in the blood due to the high amount of added simple sugars. It leads to insulin resistance and ultimate weight gain. So why do we provide special attention to carbohydrates in nutrient timing and weight control?

The ratio of protein and fats remains consistent despite the alternation in our diet because there are many benefits of fat and protein for our body. Hence, the primary nutrient that varies and alternates the metabolic process rate is a carbohydrate, an essential component for weight loss. Consuming specific macronutrients at certain times of the day can help you get to your weight loss goal faster. Timing nutrient intake can speed up metabolism, regulate hormones, and change body composition. A higher carbohydrate intake before or after exercise, for up to 3 hours, will help your body utilize the insulin and use it to help grow muscle.

There are three different types of carbs. The best time of consumption is either 2-3 hours before and after exercise- that too depends upon the intensity of the exercise you perform and some additional factors. There's a specific tolerance for carbs for each human being. While some may not feel the need to consume a lot of carbs after exercise or a long day, a lot of people won't feel stable and be distraught unless they consume a couple of happy calories or carbs. Here are the three main types of carbohydrates.

1. High in Fiber – Most vegetables and fruits, legumes, and beans. Eat any time of day.

2. Starchy – IF consuming Bread, corn, pasta, potatoes, oats, and rice. Consume within 3 hours after exercise.

3. Refined sugar – Soda, sports drinks, processed foods, fruit juice, figs, raisins, dry fruit. Treat yourself once in a while but don't make these unhealthy choices a habit.

CHAPTER 5

STEP 5: HOW TO CLEANSE YOUR BODY

WHAT IS A HEALTH CLEANSE?

A weight-loss diet is broken down into more minor elements once you pursue it accurately. Our minds mostly revert only to the part where you eat specific healthy food and leave the rest of it to luck. That's where you fail at losing weight the healthy way. There are a lot of articles on what to eat, what not to eat, and what exercises to pursue, but not even a few of those would bring the idea of taking care of your body post all the workout and restricted dieting. If you ignore yourself even after eating healthy, there's a maximum chance of the diet not affecting you, but that's what a health cleanse is for.

Speed up your metabolism and fat-burning furnace while boosting your feel-good hormones. A cleanse removes toxins from the body and restores optimal health. It benefits the entire body but mainly targets the liver, kidneys, and intestines. Cleanses typically consist of short periods of fasting, eliminating certain foods from the diet (dairy, meat, all processed foods), drinking shakes, and taking dietary supplements. You may have even seen a couple of friends telling you they've been doing a lot of cleansing or detoxing lately. That is basically what a health cleanse is. And the best part is that there is a specific health cleanse for weight loss called the weight loss cleanse.

But the primary concern of anyone struggling to lose weight would be, will it work?

The truth is a cleanse is a combination of supplements that improve the functions of your body. Many report relief from troubling situations of health conditions like consistent constipation, etc. People who undergo cleansing or detoxing also report improved moods and better energy to carry out the day. Aren't you tired of feeling drained without doing a lot of work? Weight gain is one of the most distressing health conditions that take happiness from your life. While there's a relevantly healthy amount of weight gain, constant stereotypical pressure can negatively turn the course of your life.

A health cleanse can also work for you, like improving your eating habits. It sets a pattern for your body to get hungry and consume food. That's how you feel energized throughout the day and tired by night. Your body gets accustomed to good eating habits and learns how to detox itself after the cleansing routine. How does one start with the cleansing?

Step number one to the health cleanse would be getting your food in order- learning what to consume and when to, how to give your body enough time to ingest it, and knowing when you'll be feeling hungry again. The primary notion to removing everything toxic from our lifestyle is to begin to eat healthily. So you can see how easy cleansing would be. While there's a significant difference between cleansing and detoxing, both overlap a lot of times. Many people term cleansing as the ultimate reset that puts their lives in order. The challenging part is that there isn't a single standard for all these weight loss cleanses. There are a lot of cleanses you can try for weight loss and what suits you. But the key for any cleansing routine to prosper would be consistency.

The prominent issue people with weight gain face is there isn't a single routine they can stick to. They fall into this loop of irregular eating patterns that soon leads to overeating- which is difficult but not impossible to recover from. Everyone is different in one way or another. While many overeat when they're under a lot of stress, many people lose their appetites when they face a stressful situation. So to overcome those mood swings, you turn to food, and soon it becomes an unstoppable habit. It takes a toll on your health; you get sick often, feel terrible, and have no idea where everything's going wrong- not to mention the gradual change in physical appearance and social anxiety that keep you constrained to your room. But now it's time to battle all of that accurately. Everything you've learned up until now about weight loss overlaps and seems repetitive because all of this is a fraction of each other. Everything else may spill if you try to hold it from one end only. That's why it's mandatory to master all aspects of the weight loss routine, especially the cleansing, which rounds out the rest of the elements.

BENEFITS OF A HEALTH CLEANSE

A wholesome cleanse will raise your strength level and rejuvenate and refresh you — from the inside out. It will heal you by disposing of toxins and repairing your cells. A healthful cleanse and reset will have you feeling stronger, both at the beginning stage and afterward. You need to by no means experience those dreaded starvation pains, too slow to exercise or even depart the house. Due to the human race's constant production of pollution, chemicals, and contaminants, our modern-day world is packed with poisonous materials.

And while your body is outfitted with a herbal cleansing system, its cleaning mechanisms were by no means supposed to face the steady barrage of chemicals to which we subject them. Not to mention a combination of those natural parasites and microbes we leave our bodies exposed to daily to which our immune system doesn't stand a single chance. Contaminants in the air and your food affect you more than you may think. When your physique takes in air, water, and food, it transports these fundamental elements to all components of your body so that each of your cells can use them.

Once it's finished, waste merchandise is left behind. Typically, when the cells excrete waste products, the leftover fabric is flushed away and disposed of. However, in the case of unnatural chemical substances and toxins that you aren't outfitted to deal with, the harmful substances are left to circulate and accumulate inside the body's tissues.

▶ Improved Body Functions

This is, without a doubt, the main advantage of detox cleanses. Flushing out all unsafe resources from the body paves the way for proper metabolism and promotes the perfect functioning of organs. Colon cleansing, for instance, eliminates any toxins in the intestines, improving the digestion of food and absorption of nutrients needed for the effectiveness of the liver detox system.

It's the most terrific feeling when the fog starts to lift from your mind, and you begin to feel like yourself again. A cleanse can enhance your spirits and bring back the happiness that has been buried beneath that layer of unhealthiness. It's well-known how effective vitamins and nutrients are when you adjust them in your daily routine. Choosing the right foods for your cleanse will help improve your temper and relieve anxiety, stress, and depression.

▶ Increased Energy Levels

Chemical toxins can intervene with power manufacturing in the mitochondria, the energy house of the cell.

The result is fatigue: lethargy and sluggishness. Fortunately, a detox cleanse can assist in doing away with these chemical substances enhancing electricity production.

The cleaner blood and lymph will supply nutrients from the expanded food plan to the cells and raise away the wastes allowing them to feature better. One of the first matters that human beings file after a detox cleanse is the enlargement in energy. If you've strayed from your healthful path, a cleanse is extremely good to locate your way back. Consider it a jumpstart to cleanse your body. Even a speedy five-day cleanse can bathe your cells in the nutrients they've been craving and return you to the healthiest model of yourself. The Cleanse and Reset will guide you via the method to get your fitness back on track, soften away the stomach fat, and help your body maintain itself like it naturally should.

Perhaps you want to change your lifestyle and commit to a healthy routine. In that case, a cleanse is an excellent way to get started. While you are preparing, you'll study the significance of several ingredients and their advantages to your body. Soon, you may shortly perceive which meals offer the specific vitamins you want to combat various health concerns. Your physique will thank you for the healthful reboot to your machine and cells lined with the necessities they've been craving. You'll sense yourself becoming stronger, healthier, and alive more than ever before. You'll also benefit:

- Lowering your blood sugar
- Reducing your danger of coronary heart disease
- Lowering your cholesterol

▶ Better Immunity

A susceptible immune system means the accumulation of impurities that clog the lymph- which helps transport white cells around your body to fight off any infections.

A cleanse would eliminate impurities from the blood and lymph nodes, allowing the white blood cells to move extra quickly to devour viruses and microorganisms that reason infections. Your physique will be better equipped to combat colds like the flu and other illnesses.

Allergies and other varieties of sensitiveness can additionally be improved. Our bodies are designed to detox themself naturally. But just because those structures are in the vicinity doesn't imply you are free and clear. You nevertheless want to do your share of caring for your body to hold your health. Your body can solely lift the weight for so long — trust me. When you don't assist in guiding your body's natural detox systems, you open yourself up to the threat of too many health issues, including:

- Weight gain
- High blood sugar
- A spike in insulin levels
- An increased threat of type two diabetes
- Wrinkles and first-class lines
- Heart disease

Your body works hard to strive to keep you protected and healthy. Reward it with a care-like cleansing routine every once in a while. A healthy lifestyle should be your prime motive.

▶ Weight Loss

Although weight loss is not the principal purpose of a detox or a cleanse, it can help you lose weight, tone your muscle groups and get in shape. Your body shops toxins in fats, and the body hangs on to them. A cleanse can put off the toxins that intervene with the digestive system and make you gain extra weight. Colon cleansing is a primary cleanse for making your stomach flatter by improving digestive functions. A healthy metabolism would enhance the secretion of hormones that assist in burning fats and structure your physique appropriately.

A cleanse focuses on the toxins that invade your digestive tract and threaten your health. It also gets rid of parasites and waste from your body. Your cells will be cleaned, repaired, and protected while replenishing your body with the crucial nutrients it requires. As the irritation in your digestive tract begins to limit and recovery continues, the stubborn, more incredible kilos you've been attempting to lose will melt away quickly. A protected cleanse will flood your gadget with nourishment, by no means leaving you starved. A cleanse is the ultimate support for your weight loss journey because it provides:

- Vitamins
- Nutrients
- Antioxidants
- Collagen
- Fiber
- Amino acids

- Clean protein

The elements in a natural cleanse regularly boast anti-inflammatory properties. If you occasionally feel discomfort from persistent or periodic inflammation, a natural cleanse can help limit it to an extent. The only question is how?

A cleanse limits the ratio of free radicals in your body, which, left unchecked, can lead to inflammation and, in turn, contribute to a host of continual conditions and diseases such as:

- Obesity
- Type-2 diabetes
- Heart disease
- Asthma
- Rheumatoid arthritis
- Alzheimer's and different neurodegenerative diseases
- Cancer

▶ Improved Mindset

It's the most remarkable feeling when all that brain fog goes away, the mood swings and overthinking patterns begin to fade, and you feel like yourself again. A cleanse can boost your spirits and carry back the happiness that has been buried beneath that layer of unhealthiness. Choosing the right ingredients for your cleanse will assist your temper and relieve anxiety, stress, and depression.

Have you ever suffered from brain fog or lack of concentration? Intelligence is affected simply as much by toxicity as anything else in your body. Toxins anywhere in your body, especially your colon, can be absorbed into the bloodstream and flow into the brain, the place they can affect your memory, your emotional state, and capacity to think correctly. Heavy metals present in those impurities fiddle with the production of neurotransmitters.

A health cleanse can result in extended mental clarity, concentration, motivation, and memory. It has additionally been proven to assist patients with dementia in improving their conditions. Many toxins are fat-soluble, which means they tend to gravitate toward the brain, resulting in foggy thinking. A natural cleanse can assist in limiting the buildup of heavy metals, solvents, and different toxins collected in the brain. The results? Having the readability of thinking and intellectual focal point you need.

▶ Glowing Skin

A healthy cleanse also improves your skin. Toxins can become trapped inside your skin pores, which leads to blemishes, aging, wrinkles, and dark circles underneath your eyes, distorting your appearance. As you put off the toxins, and accrued dead skin cells, you'll experience glowing, clear, and luminous skin.

The increased water intake from fruit and veggies improves pores and skin hydration merchandising supple and flawless skin. Together with zits, numerous skin issues are attributed to toxins that clog the pores and harbor bacteria which reason infections. Cleansing your body will ensure that the toxins are eliminated, and due to the multiplied immunity, the bacteria will be killed.

HOW TO DETOX WITH A CLEANSE?

Detoxification is a natural process. It's something each organism's body performs without any precise weight loss plan or specific graph – all day, each day, our body works and interacts with different organs to neutralize, transform and eliminate any detrimental supplies. When you think of harmful substances, your mind ultimately reverts the thought of any alcohol or smoking materials.

However, a clear definition of toxin denotes multiple other pollutants that can harm our bodies. Unfortunately, they are everywhere, unavoidable, and an everyday part of life; highly chemicalized products, pollution, pesticides on and in your food, pollutants determined in water, stress, pharmaceutical drugs... the list is countless.

Our body overworks to dispose of them. The liver filters 1.4 liters of blood every minute of the day. Filtering the blood requires two phases of detoxification. Phase one helps to neutralize them- this phase is where you want antioxidants, glutathione, and vitamins E and C. Phase two adds chemical substances to make the harmful stuff soluble enough. Hence, our bodies have no problem excreting them. This is where you want things like glutamine, glycine, and sulfur meals such as cabbages, broccoli, and garlic.

So, does detoxing truly work? By taking in a weight loss program that proposes the highest quality on the nutrient front than your usual, you are bathing yourself with all varieties of beneficial micronutrients that your liver needs for segments one and two of the process.

By altering our food, giving the wine and espresso a break, eating supplements, and drinking drinks that are prosperous in the vitamins and minerals that our body utilizes in the liver pathways, we're helping it combat the toxins. Giving your body a bit more to work with while lowering the stuff that slows our systems down from time to time makes you healthier and gives your body the relief it requires from the constant exhausting detoxification.

Solid meals are altered with drinks like water with lemon, maple syrup, cayenne pepper; tea; or fresh fruit and vegetable juices. There are multiple durations for different cleanses. For instance, some last a day while others are prolonged up to a month until your body is ready to detoxify on its own again. A detox weight loss program can differ widely depending on whom you ask. For some, it may additionally be regarded as an extreme cleansing diet that consists of drinking ordinary beverages for weeks on end to clear out toxins and attain healthy weight loss.

For others, the term "detox cleanse" is little extra than an advertising ploy used to shill expensive and overpriced products to health-conscious consumers. Factors like continual stress, unhealthy habits, bodily inactiveness, and a food regimen excessive in ultraprocessed foods can completely tank your body's natural detox system, making it even tougher to get rid of toxins from the bloodstream efficiently.

A body cleanse, or detox weight loss plan involves cutting out junk ingredients and increasing your intake of nutritious complete foods. A few effective detox meals can be a convenient way to assist your body and hit the reset button. Unlike other detox diets, this type of cleansing won't drain your energy stages or leave you feeling worn down. Instead, it can improve energy, restore motivation, and help you feel the best version of yourself.

There are loads of exceptional definitions of what defines the detox weight-reduction plan, or the health cleanses for weight loss. However, an exact detox weight loss plan needs to grant all of the essential vitamins your body needs while also slicing out the chemicals, junk, and delivered components that it doesn't. I know you're thinking about how to detox without throwing all of your cash in for some high-priced packages and products. Well, keep reading.

WHY SHOULD I DETOX?

The human body constantly works to dispel toxins and relies upon its organ systems to do so. Over time, it receives run down from unhealthy food choices, alcohol, caffeine, drugs, stress, and environmental toxins - part of current life. It doesn't matter how accurate or healthy your weight loss program or way of life, primarily maybe, external factors like the environment and ready-made food nevertheless require us to give our bodies recharge.

It can dispel anything that conserves us from gaining efficient fitness. When our organs are placed under too great of pressure and unable to work efficiently, this is when illness and sickness can appear. Taking time to cleanse the body and nurture these vital organs goes a long way in prevention. Additionally, it has immediate outcomes - higher energy, clearer skin, higher digestion, mental clarity, and more.

Toxins That Can Trigger Bad Health

It simply so occurs that we live in a toxic world. You don't have to know a lot to understand this barely alarming fact. The air you breathe is poisonous — not just in the town or on the highway, but the air inside your own home. All that new decors and furniture you buy comes loaded with formaldehyde and other carcinogenic compounds.

And that's simply the air. Many fruits and vegetables you buy have a thin coat of pesticide spray. Many plastics contain elements that can trigger a hormonal imbalance through smell or touch. Throw inconsistent stress and anxiety, and you're well on the road to an undoubtedly poisonous lifestyle.

That's a lot of toxic, and in most cases, it's far more than your bad overworked liver can handle. With your liver working time beyond regulation to limit and excrete these toxins 24/7, it's obtained no time for a vacation and throws a bizarre tantrum now and then. To put matters in perspective,

- Environmental Toxins
- Lifestyle Toxins
- Emotional Toxins
- Intestinal Microbes
- Metabolic Reactions

SIGNS YOUR BODY NEEDS A DETOX

▶ Stomach pain

Manifesting digestive troubles is one of the most important signs and symptoms, and it is essential to begin altering your diet. The digestive system ceases to function accurately when toxins in the body increase. Symptoms such as feeling heavy, gas, sluggish digestion, and intestinal soreness will exhibit in your everyday life.

You might also even go through nausea, mainly after a big meal. Constant constipation is one of the most significant signs that your body needs a thorough detox. After these clear signs of hormonal imbalance, you can detox your body by creating a routine to cleanse for longer periods than usual.

▶ Poor Memory and Concentration

Toxins in your body, such as monosodium glutamate (MSG) and aspartame, affect your intellect and kill the brain cells, thereby stopping the brain's oxidation. MSG is located in processed foods, and meat, while aspartame is discovered in gum, toothpaste, and sugar-free beverages.

Experiencing any of these symptoms frequently indicates that your body requires detoxification. You need to devour proper food to maintain a healthy body that doesn't need extra efforts to detoxify. Also, continue to hydrate and work up a sweat regularly.

▶ Constant headache

This kind of ache may also be extremely regular and naturally treatable, but it is a symptom that the body is no longer working correctly. If it turns into a constant struggle, go to a specialist who can diagnose the reason for it. However, even migraines are especially related to the food you eat. Avoiding greasy meals for a month is one of the first-class detox techniques to deal with headaches.

▶ Mood Swings

Mood swings manifest due to hormonal imbalance in our bodies. Toxins like Xenoestrogen are accountable for hormonal imbalance issues. To limit the degree of such toxins, you need to avoid using plastics, especially in your kitchen. With an unhealthy diet, and lifestyle choices, including high amounts of starchy carbs, sugars, and synthetic additives, the liver can make your temper change.

Suppose your body does not obtain the vital nutrients. In that case, it has very little power to finish the day, and as a result, you end up in a terrible mood. Eating healthfully and in small parts throughout the day (4-5 small meals and snacks a day) can help enhance your mood.

▶ Sugar addiction

Sugar can emerge as a dependency when your weight loss program is no longer adequate. Such a weight-reduction plan would elevate your blood sugar level, leading to a craving for extra sweet foods. Excess physique sugar is tough in many ways:

- your body stops processing the meals you devour appropriately to prioritize this "fast energy" source, which leads to gastrointestinal problems.
- Your pancreas, the organ accountable for insulin production, suffers due to the sugar excess.
- Excess sugar in the body can also motivate sleeping differences, such as insomnia.
- Change your excessive ingredients on artificial sugar for fruits while minimizing your standard sugar intake.

▶ Constant fatigue

Let's recall adrenal fatigue- if you consult a professional, they'll relate almost all types of fatigue to your adrenal glands because of the cortisol hormone responsible for stress. So, what happens to adrenal fatigue?

When your body doesn't produce the precise amount of adrenal hormones because of extra toxins, it motivates immoderate tiredness.

Also, fatigue is a primary symptom of terrible intestinal health. When the bowel no longer works as it should, it expends greater strength than usual, which is a hassle when looking to operate during the day.

▶ Skin Problems

1. Drier skin

If you don't drink enough liquids, your pores and skin gradually become dehydrated, dry, and lose flexibility. And dry pores and skin are likely to get wrinkles and age faster. Water is a fundamental thing for your body given that it is involved in many chemical tactics, and it's used via the physique in many detox processes, such as discharge via sweat, mucus, and urine.

2. Flabby skin

If you abuse meals rich in sugars and refined flours, your blood glucose exceeds. After that, some of the excess glucose affects proteins such as collagen, which inflicts skin flaccidity.

3. Grey and dull skin

When your physique has excessive toxins, your skin appears tired and loses its radiance. If you want to know how a person's feeling, you might as well observe the change in their skin tones because there's no greater indicator of health than your skin.

Generally, it lacks shine because you consume foods that genuinely no longer contribute to your health and rather deteriorate it.

4. Rashes

The skin plays a big role in the human body's cleansing processes. That's why many may term it the third kidney of the human body. It expels some of the waste components that flow into the blood through secretions such as sweat. If the quantity of toxins increases, you can note it in the look of pimples, irritations, eczema, and blackheads.

5. Acne

Chemicals and toxins that accumulate in the pores and skin are eliminated through water excretion from the body, such as sweat or urination. But irritations or zits generally appear when there is an excess of these molecules. Your pores and skin react when the liver fails to flush out the toxins from your body. Acne, eczema, skin rashes, boils, and so forth are all consequences of pores and skin attempting to remove toxins from your physique because all other organs strive to do the liver's work with the help of your skin.

▶ Fluid Retention

Your stomach will become swollen or bulging, your eyelids, lips, and arms are swollen, or your legs heavy. Again, water is your friend because liquid retention is generally provoked by an excess amount of heavy metals and salts in the body. It causes an extreme hormonal imbalance and affects your liver significantly.

▶ Alterations In Your Urine

A body with a definite amount of toxins would excrete denser urine and have a darker color. It also has a stronger smell than usual. Some might even remark it as unbearable. A simple method to assist with clean urine is ingesting one or two glasses of water as quickly as possible when you wake up each day.

▶ High Blood Pressure

Hypertension is no longer something most people can indicate or become aware of right away because they prefer going to a doctor or a specialist for those measurements. However, if you're looking for signs to detoxify your body, high BP is one.

That is why you should check it periodically since, aside from being a feasible warning that your kidneys are not working, it is a factor that increases the hazard of cardiovascular disease.

High blood stress comes from excess fats and salt, dehydration, and thick artery walls.

▶ Frequent Colds

Suppose we reflect on the thought that nearly 70% of a person's immune system is in their digestive system. In that case, we can nearly say that an intestine saturated with detrimental resources prone to flu, colds, and some diseases fly through the air each day. Consuming citrus fruits will preserve your immune system and boost in opposition to these.

▶ Insomnia

The human body adopts a simple timetable of rest. If you have problems snoozing at your common time, then there may be an issue with your hormonal balance, or rather the number of toxins present in your body may have accelerated. For instance, extra carbohydrates, caffeine, and sugar inhibit the talent feature that regulates sleep.

Even immoderate exposure to light for the duration of the nighttime can lead you to a lack of rest. Cut down on caffeine, sugar, and display screen time at some point in the nighttime, and you may sleep for longer and better.

▶ High BMI

Despite your young age and mediocre lifestyle, suffering from excessive weight gain may be due to the buildup of toxins in your body, especially if you've tried to lose weight and failed. It makes your metabolism sluggish.

▶ Stress

Stress makes the body release cortisol, a hormone that, in excess, produces problems in the metabolism. To avoid this, you can detoxify your each day activities by doing the following:

- Don't overextend your work time, mainly if you work in front of a laptop screen.
- Take periodic 5-minute breaks at work.
- Try to accomplish at least an intention a day; remember, the most minor changes count the most.
- Sleep for at least 8 hours a day. Disconnect from digital gadgets 1 hour before bedtime.

HOW DOES DETOXIFICATION WORK?

Detoxification is a term used for the process of cleansing the blood. This is accomplished by putting off impurities from the blood in the liver, where toxins are processed for elimination. The physique also eliminates toxins through the kidneys, intestines, lungs, lymphatic system, pores, and skin at some stage in the body detox. But when these systems don't work, impurities aren't properly filtered, and the physique is adversely affected.

A body detox application can help the body's innate cleansing system by:

- Resting the organs through fasting;
- Stimulating the liver to force toxins from the body;
- Promoting removal through the intestines, kidneys, and skin;
- Improving circulation of the blood; and
- Refueling the body with wholesome nutrients.

How Do You Start a Body Detox?

When starting a body detox, you first need to observe your toxin intake. Eliminate alcohol, coffee, cigarettes, refined sugars, and saturated fats, all of which act as toxins in the body and limit your recuperation process. Also, restrict chemical-based household cleaners and health care products, such as shampoos, deodorants, and toothpaste.

Another challenge to proper health is stress, which triggers your physique to release stress hormones into your system. Yoga, Qigong, and meditation are easy, and high-quality methods to relieve stress by resetting your bodily and intellectual reactions to the inevitable stress life will bring.

Keep the terrible out and get the correct in. Consume as many nutrient-rich ingredients as possible. The easiest way is to get on board with diet shakes centered on detoxifying your body. A super way to enhance electricity stages is getting a quick absorption of nutrients. This doesn't suggest that is all you are allowed to consume. Continue consuming a healthful, balanced diet, generally ingesting the foods that assist in detoxifying your physique and resetting your adrenal glands.

Detoxifying Shakes:

1. Energy Boost Shake - This morning cleanse is loaded with leafy greens and sweet apple, which will aid in the function of the liver, gull bladder, and kidneys – optimizing hormonal stability. This also purifies the blood and promotes healthy gut flora, detoxifying the body.

- -1/2 banana
- -1 ½ cups mango (cut into small cubes)
- -1 tbsp flaxseed
- -1 cup coconut milk
- Blend with ice.

2. Fat Burning Smoothie – Give your metabolism a boost with this green tea-based smoothie. High in protein, it will help keep you stay full for longer. Great for in-between meals.

- -1/2 banana
- -1/2 avocado
- -2 tablespoons of lemon juice
- -1 cup of green tea
- -1 scoop of vanilla protein powder (plant-based preferred)
- Add ice and blend it all.

3. Anti-Inflammatory Shake – As we know, inflammation within our body can cause a lot of harm and throw off our hormonal balance, causing weight gain, irritability, and exhaustion. Add this shake into your weekly routine to reduce and prevent internal inflammation.

- -half cup of Greek yogurt (plain)
- -half cup of spinach
- -1/4 cup blueberries
- -a dash of cinnamon
- -1 tbsp almond butter or natural peanut butter
- -1 cup almond milk
- Combine ingredients and blend with ice.

4. Adrenal cleanse – Achieve hormonal balance with the help of this daily shake which replenishes the nutrients the adrenal glands use when stressed.

- -1 medium-sized green apple
- -1 orange
- -1 cup chopped kale leaves
- -1/2 teaspoon ginger
- -1 cup water or coconut water

*add a scoop of protein powder (plant-based preferred) for a more filling, high in a protein shake.

- Add ice and blend all ingredients well.

5. Liver cleanse – detox your liver with these nutrient-rich ingredients for optimal liver function.

- -1 medium beetroot
- -1/2 red apple
- -1 cup cut up strawberries
- -1tbsp chia seeds
- -1 cup of water
- Blend well with ice.

6. Colon Cleanse – rid your body of that dreaded bloat with these cleansing nutrients that help boost weight loss success.

- ½ cup strawberries
- ½ cup blueberries
- ½ lemon
- 1 orange
- 1 cup coconut water
- Combine ingredients and blend with ice

OTHER NATURAL WAYS TO DETOX YOUR BODY

1. Limit alcohol intake – 90% of alcohol is metabolized by your liver. Too much alcohol can cause fat build-up, inflammation, and scarring of the liver; when this happens, the liver cannot properly filter waste and toxins from the body.

2. Get more sleep – lack of sleep is linked to high-stress levels, anxiety, high blood pressure, heart disease, diabetes, and obesity. As you sleep, your body releases toxic waste by-products.

3. Drink more water – An adequate amount of water helps detoxify your system and remove waste products from your blood. Also, it aids in digestion and nutrient absorption, lubricates joints, and regulates body temperature.

4. Eliminating or limiting processed foods and sugars – leads to numerous diseases which restrict the body's ability to detoxify.

5. Eat antioxidant-rich foods – protect cells from free radicals.

6. Decrease salt intake – causes your body to retain fluid. When salt intake is high, an antidiuretic hormone is released, preventing urination (detoxifying).

7. Eat foods high in prebiotics – allows good bacteria to produce nutrients. A change in the bacteria can cause a weakened detoxification system in the gut and leave the risk of disease and inflammation.

8. Exercise – Regular exercise reduces inflammation and allows your body's systems, especially its detoxification system, to function efficiently and protect against disease.

Positive Improvements After a Cleanse

- Improved sleep
- Improved mood
- Weight loss
- Fewer headaches
- Less bloating

- Lower blood sugar levels
- Increased strength
- Clearer skin
- Better intellectual clarity
- Better digestion

HOW TO TELL IF YOUR LIVER DETOX IS WORKING?

The liver is our most important organ because it helps our body get rid of all its toxins. Its nonstop performance helps us detoxify our blood, balance hormones, generate the bile critical to digest fat, and accumulate necessary minerals, iron, and vitamins. And when the liver does not make use of its finest function, our food, particularly fats, can't be digested appropriately. No wonder liver tends to exhaust fast, and one of the major symptoms of that is weight gain.

It is integral that you are conscious of symptoms of liver detox working as it can be used to help ease anxiety. While some signs and symptoms have to be suffered until they pass, others can be alleviated. If you think about it, all it takes are a few simple precautions. If the following signs describe your condition, your detoxification system may be attempting to tell you something.

▶ Headaches

Want to tell if your liver detox is working or not? The answer is getting a headache. It's passed off most in many instances in the afternoon and nighttime in the course of detox because you set off your physique all day long.

The biggest motive for this is that your typical daily movements have been modified. Perhaps you give up a few awful habits such as smoking, consuming caffeine, alcohol, ditching processed meals or sugars, etc. Because your body is now not absorbing these anymore, a state of affairs of withdrawal is generated and can lead to a headache.

A related motive is that you have to urinate extra frequently than standard and may also experience some unfastened stools. Both of these become major causes of dehydration in the body, which leads to a headache. A headache from liver detoxing is easier to get rid of because since it arises from dehydration- 8 glasses of water regularly will be able to alleviate it.

▶ Fatigue

Fatigue is the second highlighted sign of a successful detox, which arises from nutrient depletion and food intake changes. When your body is prompted to excrete toxins, it desires an excessive workout which isn't approachable in the contemporary lifestyle. So be ready for frequent tiredness and sleep interference. You are predicted to seem greatly fatigued. So how do you fix this rising symptom of liver detox? Take more rest than usual!

Fix your sleeping schedule firsthand. An ideal sleep is when your body has the opportunity to relax every night at 10 pm sharp – yep, just like the good old days of school. Get to your mattress with a diagram for attaining an adequate 8-hour sleep per night. While you are sleeping, your body still works towards detoxifying itself.

A little extra work that comes with liver detox is when you have to alter your sleeping schedules slightly to overcome all the sleep you've lost during the years of an unhealthy lifestyle. Taking naps is the most efficient way of getting rid of any sleep disturbance.

Complementing any extra project may additionally irritate your fatigue. Taking a reasonable each-day exercise, don't attempt to overtake it. Boosting the amount of work doesn't deliver any gain to the indispensable workload of your body in the course of detoxification.

The pressure in any form, whether or not physical, intellectual, or emotional, is inefficient.

▶ Irritability

Are you feeling more irritated than usual? Well, it might just be your body detox. Irritability is another sign of a successful body detox because your body is undergoing so many changes- it gets confusing- your hormonal patterns are altering, switching back to normal, and for this, you might experience some temporary new changes in your mood. This symptom is frequent in detoxing and is a sure sign of the recovering metabolism. Irritability, collectively with headaches, have to go away on some days and take its vicinity with the creation of calmness and energy.

▶ Nausea

You can't just change your lifestyle and diet for the better and still expect to feel the same way! The vast addition of nutrients in the body may trigger some mild nausea. To avoid nausea, you can increase your water intake, as water and minerals are best to battle nausea. In addition, you have to prevent yourself from taking pills without consuming an adequate amount of food, drinking plenty of water, and getting rest.

Nausea doesn't take a lot of your time during a detox. It can be completely gone in a few days. Though watch out for much vomiting- there might be something wrong with your stomach. Keep in mind that vomiting or extreme nausea is not a sign of a successful liver detox but rather an underlying disease.

▶ Cravings

Detoxification is the short form of getting rid of every addiction or craving your body can't handle. Especially those shots and cigarettes that are pressurizing your liver to work more than usual. You have to cut some foods loose from your regular eating regime and cut a lot of unhealthy habits out of it. But in the case of healthy body detox, you might experience some cravings. In this book, I've let you in on wholesome foods you can consume to get rid of all that starvation. Once you keep that up, you won't have to worry about the cravings anymore.

Altering lifestyle practices and weight loss plans can set off a state of affairs of transient healing. This will, in reality, motivate cravings relevant to these things you have modified and removed. For instance, take tea. If you drink it regularly and immediately revert to the option of using an alternative or skipping it, your body will miss it dearly and have you pay a little for it.

▶ Loose Stools, Consistent Urination – Upset Digestion

It's been mentioned multiple times and a well-known fact that unfastened stools and urination are two ways the physique eliminates toxins. Some of the herbs in detoxification might also be incredibly diuretic, which motivates the body to skip the water.

It can motivate a shock to the digestive system if nutrients, herbs, and extra fresh, whole meals are introduced to the stomach to get rid of those bad habits and unhealthy processed foods.

This is defined for the reason why a nutrient-complete food plan and hydration are so necessary while an entire food multivitamin is included. These will ensure that you are adding nutrients to your body. Drinking freshly squeezed fruit juices or clean vegetables and smoothies is a splendid way to aid digestion.

▶ Eczema

Eczema surely bodes nicely for your liver's detoxing capability and right cleanse. Not just unhealthy foods, but many medications and addictive materials can make the liver bog and clog. Our liver is already working hard enough to clean all the blood supply passing through it; making it work extra hard can force toxins to break through the skin, such as acne, psoriasis, and eczema. Well, they should be out of your body than inside. There are multiple treatments for skin breakouts. A whole body cleanse is the final step to glowing skin, not to mention all the healthy food you've been eating.

▶ Under Eye Darkness or Bags

Doubtlessly, puffiness suggests that your kidneys name for some attention. Kidneys, as well as livers, are two bodily purifiers. So, when you do the cleaning for one organ, at the same time, you convey positive influences on the other.

The opposite is authentic, too: mistreating one organ skill, the other is being mistreated. Moreover, the eyes always correspond to the liver. Thus, one is dealing with hassle skills the other is in trouble too. For that reason, herbs such as eyebright that preserve eyes functioning healthily and deal with the crimson eye also do the liver well. Now, you need to be gasping at the super connection within your body.

EXTRA BENEFITS OF FULL-BODY CLEANSING

When you do a full-body detox, your liver isn't the sole organ that benefits. You're also providing help to your gut, cardiovascular system, skin, and mood. Good cleanses also supply antioxidant aid to help your body shield itself from free radical damage. In different words, cleaning can be proactive and preventative!

▶ Weight Loss

Your liver produces bile, which the digestive system uses against all the fat that's been accumulated in the body. Liver cleansing is the primary route to precise bile production. Hence, detoxing your liver may be the vicinity to start if you want to lose weight.

▶ Immune System Support

If we reflect on everything, including hormonal imbalance and the function of the liver in promoting a healthier weight loss, it proposes that a healthy liver is quintessential to a strong immune system. Cleansing your liver will even provide a boost to your immune system.

▶ Discourages Liver Stones

Liver stones form in some people due to too much LDL cholesterol in the eating regimen — particularly in people with a genetic predisposition to liver stones and gallstones. The excessive LDL cholesterol makes bile harden into tiny stones, that can block the liver and gall bladder; you should even have up to 200 to 300 of these, affecting your liver's ability to detox. When you cleanse, somewhere between a hundred to 300 of the stones could truly be purged from your body.

▶ Supports Whole Body Detox

Since the liver eliminates toxins, turning them into innocent byproducts, there are commonly small amounts of toxins in your liver. It would help if you detoxed to get your liver working exactly as it should.

▶ Boosts Energy

Some of the liver's innocent byproducts are honestly vitamins the body will use. Whether they cease up in liver stones or poisonous buildup, some nutrients won't make it back into the bloodstream. When that happens, your strength levels will probably drop. Liver cleaning will make you feel better because your body will be filled with all the nutrients and energy it requires.

▶ Increases Vitality

Remember that you're restoring your liver's efficiency through the process of cleansing and detoxing. Reducing all that poisonous buildup will make your skin seem brighter and healthier. And in view that promotion of bile production helps with fat break-down, you'll additionally feel less perplexed and more relaxed.

CONCLUSION

Weight gain roots in multiple psychological disorders, including depression and crippling anxiety. This is because of lower self-esteem. How many times do you look at yourself in the mirror just wishing to swish a magic wand and immediately change into someone you want yourself to be? Or how social anxiety prevents you from enjoying your favorite foods at social events? Sometimes there's a struggle to let go of a dress that catches your eye only because it won't fit. All this can end if you devote yourself to seeking a healthier lifestyle.

A lot of dietary programs and weight loss exercising are exhausting. As discussed in the chapters of this book, an average person browses through multiple diets until they land on something satisfactory. That, too, they are prone to give up on because they're left with feeling starved and nothing more. Why does that happen? Doesn't every dietary plan showcase the aftermath of the diet- how you'll feel an hour or multiple hours post-consuming the healthy diet? The primary reason why people give up on diets is that no one lets them in on the paralyzing hunger that follows once you start dieting. So, what makes the dietary plans of this book any different?

Examining how your adrenal glands work is essential for a healthy weight loss. What good is a stress hormone for weight loss? The cortisol hormone not only improvises stress but also deals with numerous bodily functions, including influencing the metabolism.

Now stress may not be directly related to a healthy weight loss, but chemical reactions, also known as metabolisms occurring inside the human body, are. Once your adrenal glands are exhausted, they fail to produce precise amounts of cortisol in response to any type of external stressor. The result is ultimate weight gain because your metabolism slows down, and the body cannot process the food you consume throughout the day- fat accumulates around the abdomen, and you fall victim to adrenal fatigue.

In addition, you get to know your superfoods- when and what amounts to consume them in. What calories are beneficial for your health. How you'll be feeling after a single course of the diet? How much energy do these foods give you, and what changes do you experience in your physique and health. We all know in diets there is something you should avoid eating like super processed foods.

You don't have to starve to your bones to lose weight; that's what you've been doing following all those diets with a dead end. What's of utmost importance is to acknowledge that not all body mechanisms work the same. That's why you have to learn how your body works and love it for that. Weight loss is an enduring journey with its highs and lows. Nothing comes easy, but when you have the right tools, weight loss isn't a difficult thing to encounter. That brings nutrition and nutrient timings to our attention.

The role of macronutrients and when you should be eating them throughout the day is essential for a prosperous weight loss journey. But most importantly, what is it that you gain from all that except weight loss? The dietary plan explained comprehensively in this book outlines everything is not only fit for your physical health but also improves your mental well-being.

The psychological state of mind is greatly affected during the stages of irregular weight gain or provisions to an unhealthy weight loss. That is because there are multiple psychological consequences to weight gain. Depression and anxiety are the primary symptoms. In this book, you're guided to acknowledge the external stressors in your environment and how to get rid of them. Once you learn how to get rid of adrenal fatigue, you'll be able to manage stress.

Also, these healthy techniques allow you to enjoy foods that improve your mood. One of the most crippling conditions associated with weight gain is irregular mood wings- you don't know what's causing them or how to get rid of them? But now you will. This book aims not just to give you information on how to lose weight but how to improve your mental state and become the best version of yourself. Because when you feel good, you ultimately look good.

To summarize the contents, this book allows you to explore the multiple ways and methods to detoxify and cleanse your body. A Health cleanse is the best way to wind up this fitness routine because it's the terminal cherry on top. You pass the stages of acknowledging the source of your weight gain and psychological problems, learning how to fix them, eat well, be happy, and finally detoxify your body. You can enjoy not only a healthy, fit figure but also glowing, hydrated skin.

So, what is it that you do with the right tools? You use them. And on your way back to the real world, where you're more equipped than ever to attain a healthy weight loss, remember the five steps you learned to achieve hormonal stability. If you enjoyed reading this book as much as I enjoyed writing it, please take a moment to write a review of it on Amazon.

DISCUSSION SECTION

Hormonal Imbalance:

- Hormones are powerful, and they are largely responsible for many of your body's major processes. It doesn't take a significant amount to cause considerable changes in your cells and even your entire body. When hormones become unbalanced, the attributed symptoms vary quite a lot.
- In line with the speculation, we know that medical conditions that affect or involve the endocrine system in any way can bring about a hormone imbalance. However, external conflicts like stress or hormone medications can be a cause too. Hormonal imbalance leads

to a variety of complications like irregular periods, weight gain, mood swings, and insomnia. In some cases, we see that hormonal imbalances often present themself as insignificant diseases or mimic other health conditions like constipation, constant sweating, fluctuating weight, and exhaustion, causing people to disregard the importance of those symptoms and not seek professional medical help.

Signs of Hormonal Imbalance and Weight Gain:

- Statistics indicate that around 80% of women suffer from some sort of hormonal imbalance and most of them live without even realizing it their whole lives. The best way to know if your hormones are out of balance is to listen to your body. You will likely experience symptoms depending on what hormones are being produced and which aren't. Sudden weight gain is one of the most common and recognizable signs of a hormonal imbalance. While minor weight fluctuations aren't anything to worry about, gaining a significant amount of weight in a short period probably points to a hormonal imbalance.

Adrenal Fatigue:

- Adrenal fatigue, a progressively common yet often debated disease that is used as an indication of the depletion of adrenal glands, is very closely related to hormones and hormonal imbalance in general. Our adrenal glands, which usually handle the stress we experience in our daily lives, deal with it by producing hormones like cortisol — the stress hormone. As the theory goes, when people face long-term stress, their adrenal glands fail to keep up with the body's need for these hormones. When this occurs, symptoms of adrenal fatigue, such as body aches, low blood pressure, digestive issues, and lightheadedness, start to appear.

Fixing Hormonal Imbalance:

- Most studies confirm that people will
  experience at least one or more periods of
  hormonal imbalance in their lifetimes. Most
  people will be more vulnerable to this during
  puberty, menstruation, menopause, or
  pregnancy. While some may suffer irregular
  hormones continually. Although many of the
  factors that affect hormones, including aging,
  are out of your control, you can still do several
  things to balance your hormone levels.
  Common health-promoting behaviors like
  getting enough sleep, consuming a healthy
  diet of nutritious foods, and engaging in
  regular exercise may pay off greatly in
  managing hormonal health.

Treatment:

- It's important to keep in mind when seeking
  treatments for hormonal imbalance, especially
  self-medicating and so-called "natural
  remedies", as they may do harm instead of
  good. While temporary hormonal imbalances
  that occur during puberty or pregnancy are

typical, it's crucial to understand when things might be getting out of control. Stay clear of uncertified natural products for your self-medicated hormone therapy as they could increase the risk of heart attacks, seizures, and other serious conditions. Remember that there's no substitute for professional, regulated medical care. Fortunately, there are several treatment options available for hormone level fluctuations, like hormone replacement medications and anti-androgens.

Hormonal Cleanse/Detox:

- Some medical practitioners recommend a complete health cleansing for people with mild cases of hormonal imbalance. The basic principle of a hormone detox is supporting your organs of elimination, which remove waste and excretions from the body. Your body accumulates harmful substances like mercury and environmental contaminants present in foods and water. Many studies have linked these toxic substances to diseases like chronic inflammation and an overall increased risk of mortality. Although the body is designed to detoxify itself, adopting a nutritious diet and avoiding substances in food and the surrounding environment can help the organs do their job better. A good detox doesn't have to be complicated, and you can start by consuming more hormone-balancing nutrients and assisting detox function in the liver.

RESOURCES

Chapter 1

What Are the Causes and Symptoms of Hormonal Imbalance in Women? (2022)
Retrieved from: https://www.medicinenet.com/causes_symptoms_of_hormonal_imbalances_women/article.htm

Everything You Should Know About Hormonal Imbalance (2022)
Retrieved from: https://www.healthline.com/health/hormonal-imbalance

Lifestyle and Diet Can Affect Hormones (2021)
Retrieved from: https://www.healthline.com/nutrition/

how-hormones-influence-your-weight-all-you-need-
to-know#lifestyle-and-diet

Chapter 2

Adrenal Fatigue Weight Loss: How to Lose Weight with
Adrenal Fatigue
Retrieved from: https://marcellepick.com/weight-loss-
adrenal-stress/

10 Symptoms of Adrenal Fatigue (2021)
Retrieved from: https://facty.com/ailments/body/10-
symptoms-of-adrenal-fatigue/1/

How Adrenal Fatigue Causes Weight Gain, Fluid Retention and Exhaustion (2017)
Retrieved from: https://hormonesbalance.com/articles/
how-adrenal-fatigue-causes-weight-gain-fluid-
retention-and-exhaustion/

Chapter 3

36 Super Foods That Burn Fat and Help You Lose
Weight (2013)
Retrieved from: https://healthwholeness.com/weight-
loss/fat-burning-foods/

Benefits of Beetroot for Weight Loss (2022)
Retrieved from: https://prorganiq.com/blogs/new/
benefits-of-beetroot-for-weight-loss

Can Strawberries Help You Lose Weight? (2021)
Retrieved from: https://www.healthline.com/nutrition/
are-strawberries-good-for-weight-loss#strawberries-
and-weight

How to Lose Weight with Chia Seeds - Are They Effective? (2021)
Retrieved from: https://nutribolism.com/chia-seeds-
for-weight-loss/

Ginger for Weight Loss Benefits, How to Use It, and
Precautions (healthline.com)

Which Foods to Avoid when Trying to Lose Weight
(2019)
Retrieved from: https://www.medicalnewstoday.com/
articles/324564

5 Vitamins and Minerals to Boost Your Metabolism and
Promote Weight Loss (2020)
Retrieved from: https://www.healthline.com/health/
food-nutrition/vitamins-to-boost-metabolism

The 10 Best Hormone Supplements in 2021 (2021)
Retrieved from: https://happyhealthyhippieco.com/
blogs/news/hormone-balance-supplements

9 Proven Health Benefits of Ashwagandha (2022)
Retrieved from: https://www.healthline.com/
nutrition/ashwagandha

Improve Mood with Food (2022)
Retrieved from: https://mentalhealthspace.org/
improve-mood-with-food/

Chapter 4

The 3 Keys for Counting Macronutrient Ratios (2021)
Retrieved from: https://www.bodybuilding.com/
content/macro-math-3-keys-to-dialing-in-your-
macro-ratios.html

How Protein Can Help You Lose Weight Naturally
(2017)
Retrieved from: https://www.healthline.com/nutrition/
how-protein-can-help-you-lose-weight

Carbs For Weight Loss? (2022)

Retrieved from: https://www.webmd.com/diet/
features/carbs-for-weight-loss

Carbohydrates and Weight Loss (2022)
Retrieved from: https://resilient.health/carbohydrates-
and-weight-loss/

Why Healthy Fats Actually Help You Burn Fat (2021)
Retrieved from: https://maxinesburn.com/blogs/blog/
why-healthy-fats-actually-help-you-burn-fat

All About Nutrient Timing: Does When You Eat Really
Matter? (2009)
Retrieved from: https://www.precisionnutrition.com/
all-about-nutrient-timing

Chapter 5

What Is a Cleanse and Is It Safe? (2019)
Retrieved from: https://www.nursingcenter.com/
ncblog/october-2019/cleanse

10 Health Benefits of The Cleanse and Reset (2019)
Retrieved from: https://drkellyann.com/blogs/news/10-
health-benefits-of-the-cleanse-and-reset

Can A Liver Cleanse Balance Hormones? (2020)
Retrieved from: https://myersdetox.com/can-a-liver-cleanse-balance-hormones/

Full Body Detox: 9 Ways to Rejuvenate Your Body (2019)
Retrieved from: https://www.healthline.com/nutrition/how-to-detox-your-body

Made in United States
Orlando, FL
09 June 2024

47689694R00111